Sebastians
A hospital school experiment
in therapeutic education

LONGMAN PAPERS ON RESIDENTIAL WORK

*Children in Care* Edited by Robert Tod
*Disturbed Children* Edited by Robert Tod
*Therapy in Child Care* Barbara Dockar-Drysdale

LONGMAN PAPERS ON SOCIAL WORK

*Social Work in Adoption: Collected Papers* Edited by Robert Tod
*Social Work in Foster Care: Collected Papers* Edited by Robert Tod

# Sebastians

## *A hospital school experiment in therapeutic education*

Amy Sycamore

### Edited by Dr Portia Holman
Formerly
Senior Physician in Psychological Medicine
Elizabeth Garrett Anderson Hospital

Longman

LONGMAN GROUP LIMITED
London
*Associated companies, branches and representatives throughout the world*

© *Longman Group Limited* 1971

First published 1971
ISBN 0 582 42857 2

*Printed in Great Britain by
Butler & Tanner Ltd, Frome and London*

# Contents

Contents

# Foreword

This book describes in illuminating detail the work of an inspired and highly professional teacher in a hospital school. The contribution of education to therapy is seen side by side with that of psychiatry, the one enriching the other. Amy Sycamore died before her manuscript was completed, but its subsequent revision by Portia Holman, a psychiatric colleague who knew her well, would have delighted her and serves further to underline the link between the two professions.

The special significance of this experimental unit was the light it threw on the role and function of the teacher. It was not the first of its kind but probably the most articulate in its policies and aims. The chapter and verse of the daily happenings at Sebastians give ample testimony of inter-professional unity, and at the same time provide for the teacher almost a blueprint of the ideal educational environment in which to help the severely disturbed adolescent. It is not incidental that the climate of this has so much in common with that of progressive primary education, for before specializing in work for the disturbed, Amy Sycamore was herself the head teacher of a large modern junior mixed and infant school.

It was her experience here with many children so patently in need of specialized opportunity and care that led her to relinquish her headship and work with them. She brought to this work not only her professional skill and idealism but also a fearless administrative ability and considered respect for the structured setting, qualities which made her readily acceptable in the hospital in which she was employed. She knew what she wanted for her school and set about achieving it through resourceful and unobtrusive diplomacy.

It was during her years of specialized training that I had the pleasure and privilege of knowing her. I welcome whole-heartedly this vivid account of the joys, stresses and responsibilities of the

work at Sebastians, which remains a living memorial to her and
will, I believe, become a classic in the field of special education.
For Amy Sycamore was a brilliant and imaginative teacher of
adults as well as children.

EDNA OAKESHOTT

# I
# History

A pioneer scheme for the study and treatment of mental disorder in adolescence was begun at Sebastians[1] Hospital when Dr S, a psychiatrist and the physician-superintendent of the hospital, opened a unit for juvenile schizophrenics. In this hospital two wards were set aside for the reception of juveniles – about thirty boys and a rather smaller number of girls. The original intention was to admit those suffering from schizophrenia but Dr S was by no means exclusive in his selection. Since he had said: 'I want this to be a place where a child in extreme need can be given help, even if he has to be admitted at two o'clock in the morning,' there were frequent admissions of severely disturbed but not necessarily schizophrenic young people. There was, for instance, Simon, who had been shut out of the house to cool down after a quarrel with his little sister, but who came back with a chopper with which he began to hack down the back-door while he screamed out what he would do with the chopper to his step-mother. Harry had pulled down the plumbing pipes in the bathroom with his bare hands; Meg had fought the staff in the approved school, and Barty had gone out on a high girder threatening to jump to his death.

At Dr S's request the local education authority provided a teacher, who registered her first pupils on 1 November 1950. Later she was assisted by other teachers who, until the latter part of 1954, visited the children on the wards and taught them either individually or in small groups. Subsequently, a large room converted into a suite of small rooms was provided in the ground

[1] A fictitious name given the hospital to help conceal the identity of the patients.

floor of the male nurses' home. When about this time the first teacher-in-charge moved to another appointment, I was appointed to take her place in this small school in which there were three other full-time assistants. Since 1955, when I took charge, the numbers admitted were 262 girls and 320 boys, 582 altogether. Boys and girls admitted to the juvenile unit were seldom under the age of ten or over seventeen, but the majority were in the twelve–fifteen-year-old group. The numbers on roll at the end of each month varied from thirty to forty-six. The number newly admitted during a year was around seventy. Length of stay varied from under a month to several years in a few instances; the usual stay was from six to nine months.

The life of a school is influenced to some extent by the buildings which house it. The large room in the male nurses' home was partitioned off to make three small class-rooms, a staff-cum-stock room, and an office for the teacher-in-charge. A narrow passage led from the outside door. On one side of the porch was a toilet with wash-basin shared by the teaching staff and other hospital staff, and on the other was a similar toilet and basin used by all the children, boys and girls, plus visitors to the hospital on Sundays and Mondays, the visiting days. One class-room only was self-contained; the other two were separated from each other by a glass-panelled screen which could be folded back. When the screen was in position children could leave the second room thus formed only through the outer one with consequent disruption of the work going on there. In one room there was a sink with hot and cold taps and a gas-stove. The rooms were furnished with tables and chairs.

The windows in all the rooms were pegged in order to prevent anyone opening them wide enough to get out, but every endeavour was made not to lock the outside door while the children were in school, although in the early days the ward doors were usually locked. My first summer was very hot, and the tiny rooms with the pegged-down windows were dim and airless. Everything outside looked very beautiful, and the girls, who had much less freedom in the wards than the boys, begged to be allowed out into the air. On hearing that a sports club in the hospital would lend the equipment for clock-golf, I decided to borrow it and to introduce a sports afternoon into the girls' programme. They were delighted and all went off eagerly to the central stretch of closely cropped grass where the layout was prepared.

At first all went well; the play was decorous, the girls intent on their strokes. Then the young men began to appear and give ribald advice. The play became wilder and wilder, the little white ball whizzed high and fast through the air imperilling old ladies on further lawns, and the girls raced here and there with excited screams, brandishing their clubs like weapons. The staff's calls were completely ignored, and they had to pursue each girl in turn to take the weapon away and to try to retrieve the ball. Exhausted, I struck clock-golf off the list of available activities! The need of the girls for air and physical activity was not forgotten, but I longed for an enclosed garden.

The siting of the school in the male nurses' home led to a lot of trouble. Up above, nurses who had returned from night duty were trying to sleep, and down below we were trying to overcome apathy with gramophone, percussion band, and other noises. One morning, in rushed a burly young Irishman who shouted that we must keep the kids quiet! I decided to use this young man to forward my own desire to move into other, self-contained, premises. I refused to discuss the matter with him at all and told him to lodge a formal complaint with the chief male nurse. Still shouting with anger he went off to do just that and at the subsequent inquiry I supported his contention that the school was in entirely the wrong place. Later, that same young man became tutor to nursing students and was very forward-looking in patient–staff relationships and in befriending the school.

In November 1957 special school status was awarded to the hospital school, which raised my rank to that of headmistress and placed the school under the control of a Governing Body. In August 1959 a self-contained bungalow building was adapted for school purposes. The local education authority rented the school premises from the hospital, provided educational equipment and furniture, and was responsible for staff salaries.

This newly adapted bungalow was built round three sides of a small yard. Along the fourth side were the lavatories for the girls and women staff, and a covered shed, open on one side. As the water-pipes to this little toilet block passed through the open shed, a severe winter night left us without water on the following day. The rooms, however, were large, light, and airy, with a corridor on to which all the rooms opened. The head teacher's office was half-way along the corridor and almost opposite the main door from outside. We lived in a glass-house, for only the lower part of the outside wall was of brick, all the rest was glass, and from a vantage point in the corridor near the office it was possible to see into the wing at either end, and the teacher in each wing had a clear view of the other. The unobtrusive feeling of support which this gave the staff was very valuable. It was also possible to hear most of what was being said elsewhere without specifically setting out to do so, and there were gaps between the roof rafters and ceiling boards where room divisions had been made. By reason of this we all shared to an extraordinary extent in what the others were doing and could quickly move in when necessary to give aid. Yet at the same time our own territories were clearly marked out, if the children and staff wished to assert and conserve their privacy.

During the eight years under review twelve full-time assistant teachers served for varying periods; two came for a year only when secondment was granted to others to attend a university diploma course. All were qualified teachers, some were graduates, and each made a valuable contribution to the life of the school, and several received promotion when they left. The work demanded from them versatility of interest and a good cultural background, as well as the ability to keep emotionally detached while at the same time feeling a deep interest and warmth towards the children and their problems. The staffing problem was greatly affected by the fact that to begin with the school remained open for forty-eight out of the fifty-two weeks of the year, closing only for a week at Christmas and Easter and for a fortnight in June, the staff taking the rest of their leave in rotation throughout the year while the school continued to operate. If the school was to maintain an effective service, it was important that only one member of staff should be on leave at any given time, and it was felt that the Head should endeavour to keep the group of the absent teacher going. There were, however, a number of reasons against this. Twice a week admission conferences were held which the Head attended, so that any group attached to her had to be dismissed for those sessions. From time to time, too, a boy or girl was sent to a closed ward and prevented temporarily from attending school. This detention usually coincided with a strong emotional reaction, and I felt it was very important to maintain daily contact by visiting the child on the ward. No obstacle was placed in my way, but the most convenient times for the wards were during the hours when school was open; the wards were some distance from each other and from the school so that visiting in a school break left no time for the interview and no preparation time for the next period.

The most important factor against the Head becoming the substitute for the absent group teacher was that it made it almost impossible to deal internally with the strains and stresses to which the school was subjected. The ward staff had to be called in to help when the disturbance was due to something such as a fit, but I felt that it was part of the head teacher's function to be at hand, with time to give to a child who might become the centre of an emotional disturbance. Substituting for teachers on leave meant working with one group after another for a week or a fortnight and this was not long enough to permit a settled policy to be worked out with any group. It was of little value only to have the odd intervening weeks for other work.

The local education authority, after hearing these arguments, at length appointed another teacher. It was then agreed to close the school for a week six times a year. These closures were arranged to coincide as much as possible with the public holiday periods, when in any case many of the children were away. When this additional full-time teacher was appointed the staff consisted of the head teacher, four full-time group assistants and a full-time assistant to substitute for teachers absent on leave and sick leave.

Referral to the Unit was made through a psychiatrist. Many of the boys and girls had had previous treatment in child guidance clinics. Some were admitted at the request of the courts. The homes they came from presented a fair cross section of the community, for although some of them were illegitimate and had been brought up in institutions, in foster homes, or by adoptive parents, and some came from very badly disturbed families, most of them came from families which had not been broken by illness, death, or divorce and from homes where material standards and prospects were good. They came from professional families as well as from the homes of unskilled workers.

Soon after their admission each new boy or girl attended a conference presided over by the consultant psychiatrist. When the founder was in charge these conferences were very formal in nature. He and his registrars wore white coats; he addressed them as 'Dr So and So', and they addressed him as 'Sir'. We always sat in the same order: the chairman centrally, with a chair beside him for the patient, the charge nurse (male) or sister a little removed on his right, the registrar presenting the case a little removed on his left. Before him in a semi-circle sat the clinical psychologist, the social worker, the head teacher and anybody else who had been invited to attend. The registrar read through the notes; the nurse was asked about behaviour on the ward; the psychologist presented a clinical report or was asked to arrange a testing session; the social worker was questioned about the interview on admission with the parents, and the head teacher was asked about behaviour at school or was requested to admit the youngster. Then the boy or girl came in and the consultant asked questions designed to elicit the child's view of his condition or circumstances. The questioning then passed in the same order round the ring. By the time it came to the teacher's turn very little remained to be said, but a contribution was expected from everyone. Sometimes, earlier questions about home affairs had been met by muteness whereas a question on the neutral ground of school activities would elicit a response. When the child was dismissed, the reactions of the team to his personality, responses, etc., were discussed, and a programme outlined for his treatment.

A great deal of interest was being shown at this period in the relationship between the biochemical make-up of the body and mental states. All the youngsters went through a series of visits to the pathology department to have their basic metabolic rate, their blood iodine content, and other things tested, and had electro-encephalograms and psychological tests. Most of them co-operated fully in this programme, for it made them feel important. This, too, was their usual reaction to the rather imposing initial conference just described, and often a child would say to another in the school: 'You can tell her about it because she knows, she was at your conference,' quite often a valuable opening for a confidential talk. After the sudden death of the founder, the conferences became far more informal and were held less regularly, and only selected cases were given the full battery of tests. A pity, really, for the old way was a method of saying: 'We are all concerned in this with you.'

The range of intelligence in the school was wide and so was the type of schooling which had previously been received: some had attended their local primary or secondary school; some had qualified for grammar or technical schools; some had been to boarding schools, as varied as minor public schools, residential schools for maladjusted children and for the educationally sub-normal, convents, approved schools, or Rudolf Steiner foundations.

Varied, too, were the symptoms which were presented as the outward signs of their disturbance:

| | |
|---|---|
| School refusal | Enuresis |
| Truanting | Soiling |
| Sexual incidents | Encephalitic brain-damage |
| Hearing voices | Tearing clothes |
| Epilepsy | Lying |
| Hysteria | Depression |
| Rituals | Stealing |
| Tempers | Suicidal attempt |
| Noisy aggression | Delusions |
| Fire-raising | Withdrawal, etc., etc. |

The main types of disturbances seen in the school were:

(*a*) those associated with schizophrenia;

(*b*) those associated with brain-damage and/or epilepsy, with physical signs and reactions, such as fits, lack of control over particular movements, or general clumsiness, accompanied at times by whimpering and grumbling;

(*c*) gross behaviour disturbances, with general aggressiveness, fighting, swearing, running away, and stealing;

(*d*) apparently subnormal behaviour with an inability to cope socially and emotionally; and

(*e*) depressions, with suicidal tendencies.

The school served the boys and girls admitted to the hospital who were considered to be in a fit condition to receive tuition, either in the school or on the wards. Most of the children lived in the two villas set aside for them and had leave to walk in the grounds, but from time to time some were accommodated in the sick wards or the closed adult wards. All the children might be described as severely disturbed, whatever the clinical terms for their condition might be. With many of them this disturbance revealed itself as a behavioural problem, in which aggressiveness, bad language, inability to concentrate, tempers, and stubbornness might be the expression of an underlying anxiety. There were depression and apathy in some, in which a half-hearted attempt at work might be made, but the results achieved bore little relation to innate capacity. In a few the withdrawal into a world of fantasy seemed almost complete, so that scarcely any contact could be made through normal speech and action.

# 2

# The aims of the school

The first Monday morning arrived. Across the grass came a group of about fifteen girls and two nurses. Their faces were heavy and expressionless; they shambled along in a tight little clump, getting in each other's way. Many of them wore ugly-patterned print frocks, completely lacking in style, mostly far too long and tight, and with colours that had been washed down to faint blotches. Inside the building they divided into two groups and the nurses left. The girls who had any academic ability went into the further room, the rest were left with me. They went to their accustomed places and sat down. Mara went to the cupboard to get pen, paper and ink, then began to write a letter. It was well spelt and legibly written, and at first was lucid enough. But soon it deteriorated into a long jumbled list of items of underwear repeated again and again. Louise bent her face into her left breast and began to tear her frock with her teeth. Maudie laughed aloud, then drew in deep breaths, her lips pulled back into an agonizing smile. Jacquie read to me fluently and rapidly, but she could not retell what she had read. I offered to tell them a story and stood with a closed book in one hand. 'Prayers,' said Dora, pointing to the book, 'and hymns.'

'Shall we say our prayers?' and I began: 'Our Father . . .' Some hands went together and there were mumbling voices. Odd verses of several well-known hymns were being tried when the nursing escorts returned for the girls. I at least had been comforted by the reminder of spiritual help, but Maudie banged on the table and screamed, and Mara gave little Louise such a resounding slap on the face that she fell and was taken back to the ward in a near catatonic state.

The sheer misery of the encounter gave me much to think about. For one thing, the girls' clothes depressed me and must have depressed them more. In those early days boys and girls were admitted from all over the country, and for many of them visits from their parents were few and far between. In a hospital with about 800 patients and nearly as many resident staff, the provision and laundering of clothes was a very big item and only those girls whose parents visited weekly and took their things to be laundered could wear their own clothes; the others had to take what came back in the ward laundry basket each week.

The staff encouraged academic work of a formal nature, but, in the main, had to give individual tuition as standards of attainment varied from the early stages of reading and number to preparation for the G.C.E. The teachers' biggest difficulty came from the inability of the children to endure the slightest criticism or correction of their work without construing it into an indication of such deep failure that they immediately destroyed what they had done. Their inability to concentrate for more than a few minutes at a time was another considerable difficulty.

In the afternoons the grouping was re-arranged to permit everyone, boys and girls alike, to have a share in various activities which were less formal in character and which included cookery, painting, modelling, model-making, etc. Mixed grouping was customary at first, but many children withdrew completely from their contemporaries or preferred to work exclusively with a man or a woman teacher. After the move to the larger building, four full-time groups were catered for, two girls' groups and two boys' groups, in which numbers were maintained fairly evenly irrespective of age, level of attainment, or type of disturbance. This grouping was finally adopted because, in spite of differing patterns of reactive behaviour shown before admission, we found that, after admission to our community, each child who was in touch at all went through a similar cycle of behaviour of observing, testing, and finally accepting the school.

The school staff were not, of course, the only people to be concerned with the boys and girls. The doctors and ward staffs had the first and most immediate contacts, the psychologist administered tests, the social workers made contact with the families. Much happened within the Unit in eight years, including the appointment of medical registrars working full-time in the adolescent wards and the appointment of a lay psychotherapist, but it was in the school that the first attempts were made to accept the children as they were – in their illness and displaying their symptoms.

The basic principle underlying the methods used in the school was permissive acceptance of the child as he shows he is – inadequate or aggressive or compliant. In discussion, 'reflecting back' by repeating some of the words the child has just spoken, was found to be more revealing or to lead on to more discursive statement than giving 'Yes' or 'No' or using argument. Any topic of conversation was permitted and also any mode of statement, even abusive or obscene, in the hope that, when the child saw that camouflage or over-emphasis was not necessary, some idea of the real problem might emerge. Emotions shown in action were likewise reflected back in verbal statement.

Certain fixed limits to behaviour were enforced from the beginning: there must be no wilful breaking up of the furniture or special items of expensive stock; other people's work was not to be destroyed although each might do what he liked with his own; and steps were taken to minimize physical assault, although verbal aggression and acting out in other ways were tolerated.

Positive statements about progress often came from the child, who would say: 'Do you remember when I first came . . . I don't do that now' – or upon watching another child would comment: 'I used to do that, didn't I?' The staff covered relapses by questions of a face-saving nature: 'You are worried? . . . unhappy?' But as the children's self-confidence increased, the staff began to expect some response to normal social demands. The staff did not reject a child's work if he himself was pleased with it, and when some child's attitude to his work was persistently negative, teachers would take trouble to show their approval, or they would suggest that the child might welcome help and tuition.

Children who 'acted out' problems in exceptionally aggressive ways were given only one hour at school each day. When they demanded longer, they had to consider whether they could make an effort to control their unrestricted behaviour.

The plan in the school was for individual work within a group setting. The group setting showed different types of children that all were accepted. Often the activity of one child made it easy to persuade other members of the group to do something similar. From time to time there was an hour when all the children and most of the staff joined together in a communal activity to which all contributed, some by taking an active part and the rest by watching and listening. Programmes in this period included spontaneous drama, puppetry, mime to pre-recorded words, film-strips, listening to music, singing, playing on guitar or piano, dancing, and activities such as games and exercises. The day often ended with a short period when boys and girls were free to meet together in one room to play their pop records and to dance, or just to sit and listen.

A great advance was made in 1954 in setting up in its own building a school to which the children went daily, as all other children of their age group do. This helped provide an atmosphere of normality, something very necessary and helpful when many of them were asking, either anxiously or laughingly: 'Am I mad?' For some of them, it has to be admitted, school was little more than somewhere to go, providing something to do for the moment. Those able to apply themselves had an opportunity to fill in gaps, and much remedial work in reading and number was done. Some were able to explore new topics and to make progress in their former subjects; others were content simply not to lose skills they had previously gained.

Our aim was that, as far as possible, the children should come to school for the whole school-day, five days a week. Certain things had a prior claim on their time, of course: to see the doctor, psychologist, and later in our history the lay-therapist; to have tests and investigations of various sorts. From time to time other claims, not quite so legitimate from the school point of view, also intervened, but for the most part the children made a steady school attendance.

It might, perhaps, be useful here to describe the sort of rooms which makes such work easier to achieve. The first requisite is space, so that each person can make a movement, even a large movement, without touching his neighbour, for in certain moods a child will construe even the slightest and obviously most accidental touch into an act of deliberate aggression to be answered with swift and violent retaliation. On the other hand space must not be barnlike; we had one large room with a northern aspect in which two sides were almost entirely of glass. On a grey wet day the rain and greyness seemed to invade the room. The group of boys housed in it were mostly over-active, and the room was too big for its boundaries to influence them. When we moved them into a room half the size, with windows on one side only, a sort of huddling-at-home feeling began to establish itself and there was a marked change in the group.

Light in the room is very important. Children constantly worked their way out of rooms facing north into the corridor or the wing end rooms in search of the sun. The height of the windows matters too. Supervision of these youngsters must be constant but not obtrusive. From low placed windows the staff could see what was happening to children who ran outside. It is equally true that the youngsters could also see everything that happened outside, but distracting and annoying as that sometimes was, it was even worse if the staff felt shut-in while activities unseen but guessed at went on outside.

So the room must be large but not huge, light, and with a view on to its immediate surroundings. A built-in store cupboard or storeroom with a good lock, and a deep sink with hot and cold water are essential – and a small cooking-stove is invaluable.

At Sebastian's, after the 1959 move, only one group was without a built-in store room. All had sink and water; two of the four had a gas-stove. In addition, each room had at least one cupboard which could be locked. The locks had to be renewed time and again, but these cupboards enabled the teacher to put into safe-keeping treasured objects brought along or made by the children and to put things away or bring them out accordingly as he wanted to narrow down or to stimulate interests at any given time. It was the teacher who decided whether, and when, the cupboards were left open and how much free access was allowed. More often than not they were left open but control was in the hands of the teacher and not of the most dominant child.

The rest of the furniture was made up mainly of tables and chairs; the tables were of several sizes and most of them were topped with formica and were easily cleaned after use. The chairs had to be strong. Along one side of the class-room was a fixed bench top where items could be left out on display if desired and where a child could safely stand or lie out of the way of the room's general activities. Open spaces in the class-room should be clearly defined, so that a child who is seen to be cramped up or to be intruding too much on others can be drawn to a more spacious area. As much as possible should be going on in the room at the same time, a multi-purpose room, with the teacher's eye over all. If the floor can be easily mopped down, so much the better; for clay, plaster of Paris, cooking materials, water, etc., will all find their way on to it however carefully spilling is guarded against. And no one must be heartbroken at finding that it is not practicable to keep the floors highly polished and shining, as it is the joy of hospitals to do.

A very important requisite, too, is that the room shall be self-contained and have quick and easy access to the outside of the building so that the comings and goings of any one group do not disturb the others. We learned this the hard way during our five years' occupation of the old school. It was helpful, too, to have a glass panel in the class-room doors so that the Head could keep visual contact with the other teachers and find out what some of the noises within meant without actually entering the room.

## PERMISSIVENESS AS A POLICY

The school, although housed in hospital premises and ancillary in purpose to the Unit, was provisioned and staffed by the County Education Authority and formed, therefore, part of the County's special school system. The course followed had to be approved by the authorities, but primarily it had to be one which the staff felt was of benefit to the boys and girls, not merely ultimately in some distant future but in the here and now of their problems and distress. Long before their admission to the Unit many of the children had called attention to themselves by difficult or strange behaviour at home, at school, or in the community at large. Some had attended child guidance clinics, some had been sent from home to special boarding schools and some had been before the courts and possibly held at remand home or approved school. Many had moved from foster parent to foster parent, others had roamed the countryside and been exposed to physical and moral danger. A few had withdrawn into a world of fantasy, or had become mute and uncommunicative.

Our first task was to decide what were these children's greatest needs. In spite of the varied diagnoses of the children, we could see that at some point in their history they had suffered, or felt they had all suffered, deprivation and rejection. Some case histories showed this startlingly clearly; in others the family, real or substitute, appeared to have shown great concern and care, yet to the child this concern had no value because of the lack of an indefinable something essential to the establishment of his identity. This gave him a feeling of hollowness, of being outcast and unloved, and some youngsters who were suspicious and lonely shrank from any human relationship in case they were to experience again the pain of being rejected. Others fought against this feeling, shouting down the possibility of abandonment and building up for themselves a spurious feeling of well-being by continual activity and self-exhibition. It seemed to us, therefore, that the new community to which they had come must provide a place in which they dared to explore feelings of these sorts and in which, in spite of their behaviour, they could find a measure of acceptance.

Obviously, as the setting was a school, a school framework and machinery had to be used. Almost all the children had been to other schools (some to a large number of other schools) and had a pretty clear idea of what 'school' meant in terms of programme. Since some had had painful experiences at a former school, with a specific teacher or particular activities, since others had refused altogether to attend school and others had been expelled, they came to us with built-in antipathy and open antagonism. Many, however, had seen their earlier schools as part of the normal way of life and had made reasonable progress. All of them on arrival to us were welcomed and placed in one of the groups. Some settled down at once to work, confident that in so doing they could not go wrong; the others idled or flatly refused to give attention.

It did not take long for the message that we were prepared to like him or her to convey itself to each child, and for each to begin to respond in a way typical of him or her self. The cautious, suspicious children withdrew still further; they had been caught by niceness before, mistaking it for something deeper and had no intention of falling into that error again. The more outgoing children relaxed and a few were able to live quietly with us from that point onwards, salving their wounds and making their own recovery.

The more damaged children of an outgoing nature began to test the situation, saying in effect and indeed sometimes saying in words: 'You say you like me. I will show you what I am like, and then see.' A good deal of what they showed was unpleasant, and by normal standards intolerable; that is to say that if, in addition to providing academic work, the staff had thought its primary purpose to be the inculcation of socially approved behaviour, they would at once have disciplined these children, but the primary purpose was to re-establish in them a hope that life was worth living and, only after that, to try to bring them to what we believed were more desirable ways of living it.

It may be felt that the staff were taking too strong a view of their primary purpose by imputing these very violent feelings of distress and despair to these boys and girls. Not all were sufficiently articulate to express their feelings except in their outrageous behaviour, but read these extracts from fragments of unprompted writings that have survived:

BERNADETTE: Oh Death is a way out of this hell.
 I cannot tell.
 O for some peace of mind.
 They could be kind.
 I want to find a valley of peace by myself
  All alone
  Like the sea foam.
 My life is all hell.
 I'd love to tell.
 There must be a way out of it
 Like a star is lit.
  Death is a night
  That is full of fight.
 O life is too cruel for me,
 It is like a suffering tree.

 The hell of a life I cannot bear.
 It isn't that I do not care.
 If only people understood –
 I'd like to live, I know I would.

MAURICE: The cinema will show its lights again,
 The fire will glitter around the hearth.
 But I'm afraid, Gillian, my lights are gone;
 I'm alone in the dark, without any guiding hand.

JANETTE: I feel like a worm all screwed up down below;
 I feel like a corpse cold in the mortuary;
 I feel like an embryo as yet unknown,
 Or like an atom lost in eternity.
 And yet I want to feel loved and warm.

ANDA:      'Once upon a time' stories mostly start.
How I wish I too could write one
Out of the clear air, out of space,
Fantasy, pretence, overwhelming me,
To the heart of things.
A secret, a creed, to me,
Known by none other,
Beyond price,
A reason for a life worth living
In excitement,
Worth one single try
Sometime, perchance, to see the truth in me.

One girl, who made particularly attractive charcoal sketches, conveyed her feelings not only in the pictures themselves but in the captions she added, some of which read: 'Why am I always the outsider? Running away again? We don't want YOU, we hate, hate, hate.' They seemed, too, to show their despair in the abandoned, dare-devil way in which some of them climbed to high places, jumped and hurled themselves at things, oblivious of the danger and resultant pain. Elizabeth was one of several who showed complete unawareness of weather conditions, staying out in just a light frock in pouring rain, sitting on the ground in snow, standing for a long time by the side of the building in a keen wind when everyone else sought to be inside to be warm. Terry, Babs, Val, the list could be extended to a great length, wandered off into darkness, loneliness and hunger. Several took active measures to inflict injury on themselves: Jeannette set fire to a curtain, wrapped herself in it and sustained extensive burns; Saidie swallowed pins and needles; Katie broke windows then tore her flesh on the jagged edges; and attempts were made at self-strangulation and other forms of self-mutilation. Not all such incidents were suicidal in attempt by any means, for some, more in the nature of hysterical demands for attention and help, were staged where rescue was at hand but, nevertheless, they were desperate enough.

When, therefore, these children proceeded to test the reality of our acceptance of them, we had to respond by behaving in a way which seemed loving even to their distorted way of looking at things. This was not easy for teachers who expect certain patterns of behaviour in the relationship between juniors and their seniors. We were uncertain whether we would be able to do without punishments to emphasize the limits we set to the children's behaviour. Yet to these damaged children punishment meant that we stood against them, not with them. As Stephen had said: 'Your friend was going to be your foe.' On one occasion Lisa, who had very little control, was constantly admonished to follow the programme which had been prepared for her, and at the end of the session she looked at me sadly, her blue eyes brimming with tears, and said: 'All the afternoon you have been saying "I hate you, Lisa".' I could well have justified my action by all the usual arguments, such as that giving in to children is to spoil them, that they came to school to learn, and that a teacher is there to teach. But what Lisa needed to learn at that moment in her development was that she mattered, that we could tolerate all her tiresomeness and inattention. Love had to be seen by her to be love in the terms in which she was capable of understanding it, as unlimited response to her demands, the giving to the point of spoiling, not the exercise of power. She was not yet able to appreciate that love given also makes demands. G. H. Mead in *Mind, Self and Society* puts forward the idea that the original sense of identity in a child is made up of the attitudes, words and gestures of others towards him; he sees himself mirrored as it were in what they give back to him. So on that particular afternoon Lisa perceived herself in my reactions to her, in my authoritative voice and stern face, as an undesirable no-good, and this she was not able to endure.

The word permissive has already been used in connection with the staff attitudes in the school. It is not, perhaps, a good term, for it is interpreted by many people to mean licence and lack of discipline. But discipline and control were our aim, they were the goal towards which we hoped the children would travel. Before taking the hospital post, I had worked in, and administered, other schools, with 'normal' curricula and methods of discipline, but the children who came to the psychiatric hospital needed something different. They needed to look at their own feelings and reactions, to look at the circumstances which had brought them down into the deep ditch in which they found themselves, to look back at what they could recall of people and incidents earlier in their lives, and eventually to look forward to what they could bring to life and to what life could offer them in the future. This intensive looking could only be done in a place apart from the ordinary pressures of daily living, in a safe encampment where time could appear to stand still for a while, or even run backward, and this we sought to provide. The term should, therefore, not be just permissive and should imply not a withholding of judgement, but a withholding of condemnation. We did not depart from our standards and values, but waited hopefully for the children to choose to make them their own. We believed (1), that the children had the ability to make a good judgement, and (2), that a right perspective could be established so that it would be their wish to live by their good judgement. This was the creative power in the method and this more than compensated for such temporary confusion as occurred.

The behaviour that we had to tolerate included pinching, punching, pushing and biting. These were some of the ways in which they showed anger, rebellion, and hatred. Of course, such acts had to be restrained; other children had to be protected, and the staff could not be called upon to endure this sort of thing indefinitely, but the restraint had to be accompanied by explanation, not punishment; by telling the children that we liked to have them there, and by some interpretation of why they felt like acting so. An outburst might be due to jealousy over someone else being talked to, or to frustration over failure in a task, or to an upsurge of unhappy feelings because there had been no letter from home. We had to find ways in which they could discharge aggression that would not leave a hang-over of too great anxiety, for assaults against people were followed by great waves of remorse. This was especially so if the assault was not answered with anger, for an angry response created something almost tangible to fight against and was seized upon illogically as justification for the original assault. We provided a punch-ball and so great were the attacks made upon it that twice the metal retainer for the spring broke. Sometimes the assailant marked a face on the ball. 'That is my old man,' or, 'That is the P.T. master at my other school', and bruised knuckles testified to the hatred felt for that person. Sometimes someone hung a figure made of straw from the rafters and punched and stabbed and finally lynched it, or a pillow of straw would be punched and kicked. Pianos and drums were played furiously, and lumps of clay banged into submission, sometimes with a verbalized comment showing whom it represented in the child's thinking. A chair would be thrown down, a cup or basin smashed, a table up-ended to overturn what it held, a window would be broken, or a door kicked. While we preferred these to assaults on people every effort was made to conserve furniture and preserve the fabric of the building, and we usually pointed out some of the consequences that would be bound to result – we should be short of paint for a week or two, no cups would mean no tea, we might have to pay for the replacement of the article destroyed. The best thing was for the consequence to arise naturally from the destruction, but this did not always happen sufficiently quickly to be effective. An example of direct consequence was seen when cooking ingredients were given out. Each week each child was entitled to a supply of ingredients, limited by the amount of money which could be spent on this one activity, and one egg was included. If in an outburst of temper or an excess of hilarity the egg was thrown and broken, that child's cooking for that week was perforce limited to making pastry or some other concoction which could be made without using an egg.

From time to time fighting broke out between two boys. If it were preceded by tense, white-faced preliminaries, it could often be resolved by one of the women staff walking between the boys and asking to be told what had gone wrong. The boys would ask her to get out of the way in case she got hurt; usually she stayed, and, because of the ingrained belief that boys and men do not hit girls and women, some other way of settling the dispute would be agreed on. If a man tried to intervene in this way it usually precipitated the fight. Often, however, there were no preliminaries. An apparently quietly working group would be suddenly torn by two boys grappling in deadly earnest with no attention to rules. Mostly other boys refused to get mixed up in it but sometimes a more responsible member of the class would join with the staff to separate the fighters before real damage was done and, occasionally, if there were only women staff in the school help had to be sought from the ward staff. It was often found that these fighters were quiet, self-contained boys who did not use other outlets for aggression. Another way of deflecting the uncontrolled fight was to insist that, since there was not enough room inside for fighting, the combatants must go outside on to the grass. Once outside, either the battle became a friendly tussle or the one with the quickest legs would make his escape.

The girls' battles were usually verbal ones and they used

techniques of ganging up to ostracize another girl but, when there was a pitched battle, everyone had to use every effort to separate them for they went for each other's faces, hair, and eyes, and had to be held immobile until the tension resolved in tears. Staff had to watch out for themselves as best they could, for there were no inhibitions here when the fighting stage had been reached. Being allowed to go outside was a way of reducing many tensions. Sometimes the youngsters burst out, as if part of an explosion. When the school was in its early small premises, and the wards were for the most part kept locked and the school windows were pegged, we kept the school door unlocked and permitted children to sit on the steps and on the grass outside. We ran the risk, of course, that they would go beyond recall, but they seldom did. In the second building some of the windows had lower panes that lifted out completely and, if the door were closed, the windows were used illegally as ways in and out. One boy who had been a school refuser was told he might leave whenever he wished, but that it would be appreciated if he came and indicated that he was about to go. He exercised this privilege fairly, saying that at times he felt that if he stayed he would go 'mad'.

Certain risks had to be taken in this sort of relationship with the children and it was essential not to show fear in a tricky situation. If an adult showed fear, the child saw himself as indeed a bad person. But if the adult could live through the dangerous situation fearlessly, the child saw himself as potentially the master, not of the adult, but of his own aggression. Keith was asked to return a record which he had snatched from one of the girls. He put it into his jacket and spread out his empty hands, but the record slipped down and I picked it up, whereat he immediately punched me on the arm. I merely commented that I would return the record to the girl. The next day I showed Keith privately the bruise on my arm and wondered if he knew that he had such strong hands. He brought another boy in later, and said: 'Show him what you showed me.' I refused, saying that it was a private matter between us. A number of times during the next few weeks he would say, quietly: 'I hit you once, didn't I? I don't do that now.' Actually he did a lot of damage with his strong fingers and sometimes hurt animals, but this incident between us enabled me to speak to him openly on these occasions without fierce and guilty resentment preventing him from listening.

As a woman head teacher I represented different things to different children: to some the mother, to others authority, and to others the witch. One boy remarked that I was kind and smiling, then added: 'But how do I know that behind it you are not a witch?' and he painted a series of pictures of witches. A small coloured boy who had been the despair of several institutions used to vent on me the anger aroused in him by other people and events of which I knew nothing. He would appear in front of me armed with large stones or swinging his buckle-ended belt. On one such occasion we faced each other in the school-yard for several minutes, an endless time, watched by other children and staff who feared that a move on their part would harm me. Finally a boy got out through a back window, came round behind the angry boy and disarmed him. Already his anger had passed and danger with it, but there was also the problem of losing face, but the other boy resolved that, too, when he removed the brick. Sometimes aggression towards the staff aroused such guilty feelings in other children that they attacked the aggressor, who then had to be protected against them. Each member of the staff was seen as a provider, but was also a central figure to whom gifts could be given; he or she was looked to to give love and was also there to be loved.

We realized that we were not significant to the children as teachers, but as substitute parent figures, and that much of what we were called upon to endure showed the extremely ambivalent feelings that they held, often unconsciously, towards their parents; feelings of hostility and loving, alternating indeed, but often expressed in one and the same act. Something of this sort may have accounted for Rob's behaviour when on three separate occasions he made his way into the school when it was closed and left his faeces. The first time he went into the large room used for the gramophone session and hid the faeces in a coloured cardboard box in a drawer; on the other two occasions he got into the staff-room and deposited them, once in a box of shiny brown conkers under the table and, another time, in a box of apples. At one level he was being very aggressive, at another he was making a gift. The cooking ingredients were kept in a large cupboard in the staff-room because the staff-room door was locked each night, yet once or twice a term we would arrive in the morning to find that the room had been broken into, the cupboard rifled, leaving an indescribable mixture of sugar, margarine, flour, eggs, treacle and jam, spread over the floor, walls and chairs. School attendance for everybody would have to be postponed until the mess had been cleared up and there could be no more cooking until the next restocking of the cupboard. Here again, this need to spoil and squander food-stuffs seemed to indicate their trust that the parents would provide, and a desire to hurt them by destroying what they provided.

The children hated the school to be closed, yet they sometimes inveigled their teacher into going outside so that they could barricade the room against his re-entry. When this was reported to one of the other teachers, he or she generally asked one of the more responsible in the room to see that no damage was done. This brought the matter on to a level of mischief instead of hostility, and the affair was usually over in a very short time. It was essential, however, that these incidents should be infrequent and the staff had to be continually alert to forestall such out-manœuvring. Sometimes the children would try to organize a strike. For a time the play would be acted out, with manifestoes and demand notes issued to the head teacher from a headquarters outside the school. Gradually, however, the rebels would move inside, and the strange situation would arise that the literature of the rebellion became a school project. For a little while, its life would be continued in posters and wall slogans, but before long the school programme would envelop them again. The principal thing was not to lose touch, but to accept these demonstrations as the working out of a problem (not necessarily the overtly stated one of anti-school activity).

The attempt to shut out the teacher by striking against co-operation in a work programme, the destructive play in the food cupboard and other incidents of this nature were all demonstrations of rejection from children towards the staff which may have had two purposes. One has been discussed – to test the sincerity and trustworthiness of our affection by displays of 'badness'. The other perhaps went something like this: the child had felt rejected and had found this condition unsupportable. Then, on reflection, he began to see that rejection is not necessarily absolute and devastating. It might be something which everyone has to experience and must learn to tolerate. After these escapades we found that some of the perpetrators had become less vulnerable and were able to take the risk of making relationships.

This desire of the children to test the staff's tolerance of rejection, might account for some of the absconding that occurred from time to time, especially after the régime on the wards had become more permissive. The old plan of dealing with returned absconders, whether they came back at their own volition or were brought back in a police car, had been to confine them for a time in a locked ward, with all privileges stopped, including school. But the newer method was to hold them within the family of the Unit without being punitive, although for a while they might only attend school and other social activities outside the ward with a nurse to escort them from door to door.

On the whole very little absconding took place from the school itself, but it sometimes occurred on the way to school in the morning or on the way back to the wards in the afternoon. Sometimes it seemed to be nothing more than a reaction to boredom, a desire to have something different from the uneventful routine of a self-contained hospital. In some cases it was an act of initiative, a useful sign that timid submission had been conquered, but on the whole the absconders, particularly the girls, felt a good deal of anxiety, even girls who might have sought such danger had they remained at home. When, after 1958, the catchment area of the hospital became smaller, it was often found that the children ran home. Then parents and doctors conferred, often with the result that the absconding was turned into permitted leave followed by voluntary return. Sometimes the running away would call a family's attention to the bleakness of the child's situation and the family ranks would close round the child to reject the hospital.

Most of the time, rebellion and testing out were frequently shown in the unorthodox use or misuse of materials. To keep to a minimum the disorder arising from this, and also to conserve stock, only small amounts of expendable materials were made available at a time: a teaspoonful of powder paint of each colour required was given, just about enough plaster of Paris powder for the projected model, the cookery tin in each class-room contained one jar of sugar, one bag of flour, etc., two or three pieces of balsa wood were given, all with the promise of more should the need arise. The children knew that materials were there and that they could have them on request for proper purposes. Even with these limitations the children achieved much messy satisfaction. They painted on windows and walls, and on any blank space that offered itself they wrote slogans whose wording left much to be desired. Often the children were concerned with writing their own names, high up in places beyond the reach of anyone wishing to rub the names out, so that sometimes they even used the ceiling for this purpose. They never tired of making statements of love and hate, or of expressing fears in slogans. Children who only dared to rebel anonymously put up odd words surreptitiously. Those who disliked what they saw on the walls cleaned them from time to time, and others did so now and again as an act of restitution. After a child had made a mess, he was asked to help in restoring the room to a good condition. An answer to the effect that the cleaner could do it at the end of the day would lead to discussion of the part played by each member of our community and the respect due to each. We were extremely fortunate in our various helpers, two of whom stand particularly firmly in our affection – Bill and Glad. They had a thankless job in that the place they tidied up each day was doomed to untidiness at the beginning of the next day, but they were able to see the children's needs and motives. The children also were quick to know this and in time began to feel affection which led them to do much to restore order before they left.

In short, the aim of our 'permissiveness' was to help the children to see that we were not offering them unrestrained licence but wished them to find out about themselves and learn to apply their own restraints. Some of them found this very difficult and much more painful than submitting to external punishment. When they were not opposed with criticism and anger, they found their own anger evaporating to reveal a residue of unhappiness; they had a sense of fighting in cotton wool instead of assaulting a brick wall and began to understand that the brick wall they were expecting was of their own making. Many of them went on to realize that a changed way of thinking would result in changed relationships. To some this was intolerable, and they would have preferred a punishment which would absolve them from giving further thought to their predicament. Panic against having to make a choice which might lead to change often made a child beg: 'Tell me off . . . give me the cane.'

The use of bad language was one of the most easily noticed departures from the customary behaviour of pupils in a school and we even had complaints that the children were being taught to use bad language. Incidentally, these complaints often came from adults whose own mode of speech was not above reproach.

The fact was, of course, that most children in this age group have already acquired a vocabulary of swearing and the boys and girls who came to us knew quite well that they gave offence by using this vocabulary in the presence of certain people.

In the main the use of bad language served one of two functions. Bad language was used by some as an instrument of attack, to wound through shock or annoyance. Directed at the dignity and position of the hearer, it was thrust in like a sword to deflate or dismember. It became a mark of the rebel who was refusing to be overawed and to remain quietly insignificant. For others it was a magic device which gave them a feeling of power in themselves and bound the power of the environment. Often these children were somewhat uneasy about it themselves, and contented themselves with uttering an initial letter instead of the whole word.

It was not necessary for the staff to know what purpose it was serving before making an attempt to deal with it, for deal with it they did, in spite of opinion to the contrary, but their method was in line with the general principle of letting growth and control spread from within the child, and, therefore, its effect was slow and not readily apparent. A useful technique was to reflect back, by using the child's words. This does not mean that bad language comparable to the children's was used back at them or used indiscriminately in general talking – in fact the staff observed a high standard of polite speech – but the child's own phrase was repeated to him, prefaced with 'You think . . .' or, 'You have just said . . .' Milly was a particularly explosive girl, who on arrival at school would appear at the door of the office, put out her tongue, and say 'bitch' in a loud voice and then go on to her class-room. After several mornings of replying quietly, 'Good-morning, Milly,' I made an opportunity one day when she came in to ask for a book, to say: 'I think you feel cross with me when you come to school because you call me bitch.' She ran from the room and said to her teacher: 'That naughty lady in there said "bitch",' and she went into peals of laughter repeating again and again that I had said 'bitch'. The next morning she again used the term, but her eyes twinkled, and in a few days she gave it up. Similarly Grace, who produced plays, poems, and stories at a great pace, brought in a play and asked me to read it with her. In the part assigned to the head teacher came F . . . I asked Grace what this stood for, as the person in the play appeared to be brave enough to say other things. After some hesitation and with a look of great daring, she wrote in the missing letters, and I read the sentence in full. The effect was immediate: she, too, rushed from the room, laughed loudly, and told everyone that I had used a bad word. Her teacher pointed out that it was her word, used by a person she had made and that she had chosen that the Head should have that part to read.

Using the reflecting back technique seemed to show that, as a weapon, bad language could be made harmless to its intended victim and, as magic, it was powerless if its secret was understood. For some children, of course, the use of bad language was a lazy habit which continued after its significance had been lost. They were challenged on this point, particularly when they were wanting week-end leave or talking of discharge, and they were encouraged to show their increasing control by cutting out un-desirable language. It was sometimes noticeable, however, that some, after a period of leave, indulged in more bad language than usual. Presumably it indicated something of the strain that still existed in their home relationships. It became apparent, too, that the use of bad language was as much a personal, individual matter as any other symptom. Many children in the school were com-pletely unaffected by it and never used it.

There was another language apart from the spoken language to which we paid great attention, and that was the language of mood, the interplay of small reactive gestures that gave the colour of a child's thinking, straws which pointed like signposts. One of the chief of these was a hollow gaiety – not the relaxed overspilling of happiness, but a brittle laughter that was only a sound, or a shaking, hysterical compulsive chuckling that covered panic, or an urbane empty smile, or a cruel derisory glee. A number of these mechanisms employed by the children were barriers, and this laughter barrier was one of the most impene-trable, for it was the deceptive outer guard of a number of barrier devices and, as in the old fairy stories, when the saviour-hero had picked his way through pleasant places designed to divert him from his purpose, the attacking swords of open hostility still had to be faced. The smiling children were, it seemed to us at times, the most deeply despairing, but they covered their despair with a mask and dared not let even themselves know what was beneath the mask. St Catherine is said to have urged her followers to know their tears. In Hans Andersen's story of the *Snow Queen*, Gerda's warm tears release the frozen-in Kay:

> 'She wept bitterly and her hot tears fell on his breast and thawed the ice and penetrated to his heart and washed out the splinter of glass . . . Then Kay burst into tears. He wept until the glass splinter floated into his eye and fell with his tears. Then he knew his old companion.'

In Kingsley's *Tom and the Water Babies*, it is old Grimes's tears that break down the imprisoning chimney stack:

> 'As poor Grimes cried and blubbered, his own tears . . . washed the soot off his face and off his clothes; and then they washed the mortar away from between the bricks; and the chimney crumbled down and Grimes began to get out of it.'

Also, in Paul Gallico's modern fairy story *Love of Seven Dolls*, tears reveal the salvation of Capitaine Coq:

> 'Mouche felt the trickling of something warm over the hand that held the ugly, beautiful, evil, but now transfigured head to her, and knew they were the tears of a man who never in his life had yielded to them before, who, emerging from the long nightmare, would be made forever whole by love.'

In the upbringing of our children we tend to teach them that tears are babyish, that boys and men must not cry, that at all costs one must preserve an outward show of well-being. If babyhood's reactions are not outgrown and if our inner being is ill, this teaching is harmful rather than helpful. Sometimes, particularly among the children who had psychotic symptoms, the tears never came, even though the face puckered and crying sounds were made. When a child was able to drop his barrier of laughter and let the tears come, then something was swept away comparable to Kay's glass splinter.

We had to learn to recognize the deep grief of this group and give it opportunity for expression. The group conditions under which we worked made it possible, sometimes, to make an apparently casual approach, for anything like a frontal move would be too dangerous and too cruel; but another child's comment on the laughter or the smiles enabled one to ask, whether some people laughed instead of crying, or to say that, if they cried instead of laughing, perhaps their crying would never stop. Our attitude to other children's tears showed them that we did not despise people who cried: we did not pester them to know why they were crying or try to jolly them out of the mood. It could be seen that moods were respected as were mechanisms adopted for releasing too high tension and the discharge of deeply repressed feelings.

It must be remembered, in reading this account, that many of the children we were concerned with had been subject to the normal pressures of upbringing in family, school, and the wider social community, but they had made a response other than the usual one and, therefore, if they were to be helped, special methods were called for. In the 1957 Willson Lectures given at the Southwestern University, Texas, Dr Carl Michalson stated:

'Christians are often scandalized by psychotherapists who seem to relax the moral standard in order to relieve their client's anxious guilt . . . There is not a single value to be conserved by exacting standards of behaviour for which the emotional and spiritual conditions of achievement are lacking. Moral flexibility may not in itself be healing, but it does less damage than the tightening of the demands that are already cracking one's nature.'

We did not claim for ourselves the title of psychotherapists, but our hope was that we might contribute an environment which provided the emotional and spiritual conditions for achievement.

All sorts of causes and reasons, differently described by different schools of psychology, lie behind the behaviour and reactions exhibited to us in the school. It has not been the purpose of this book to try to sort them out nor to give support to any one view rather than another. We saw the damage done by fear of failure, and consciously sought to encourage a mode which might further creative achievement.

But there were times when, in spite of our belief and knowledge, we ourselves made mistakes, because of our emotional reactions, because of pressure from others who did not share our aims, or simply because of tiredness. We often did the wrong thing but, sometimes at least, we saw what we were doing and tried to put it right. There was a locked filing cabinet in the office and a spare key to it was kept hidden in a desk drawer. One day a girl came into the office, found the spare key and was discovered looking through the contents of the filing cabinet. On inquiry, it was clear that a member of the staff had left the office door open. I spoke to the girl telling her that in future she must knock and wait for permission to enter, even if others were coming freely in and out of the room. That evening, on thinking it over, I realized that the other teacher had been somewhat irresponsible but I had found it easier to act against the girl than a colleague. The next morning I called the girl in and explained that I had acted unfairly. She was amazed, and said: 'Why have you changed your mind?' When I tried to explain that I had made a mistake and was now acknowledging it, the girl replied: 'I think it is a miracle.' On other occasions, too, we found that if a member of staff could admit to a child that he had behaved badly, the child could bring himself to admit to faults on his side.

There were certain aspects of our policy which we had to be constantly reviewing. Someone would, for instance, advocate allowing regression, so that a child could return to a known safe point and grow up again from there. The question was would he grow up, or would he stick there? Some, of course, were in a regressed state when they were admitted: were we to give them sanction to stay there? All of them, however sick, had showed some normal behaviour. We worked normally with them in these areas, and, as it were, waited with them for the day when they would show that they no longer had need for the abnormal or regressed behaviour, but were prolonging what was now in effect a bad habit. Among our notes is one on Rosa that reads: 'Today she stamped near my feet but not on them, and I have decided from now on to reflect back to her that her tempers are no longer compulsive.' Another girl, Pamela, who used to have sudden, severe outbursts in which she threw things around and smashed things up, rushed into the office one day saying that she would break up our new and expensive globe. Instead she picked up a small tin containing pins and clips and threw that down. When she was calmer, I put it to her that she was now giving into herself unnecessarily and that the time had come for her to find a more grown-up way of expressing annoyance. With her understanding and consent, a programme of sanctions was worked out. For some time we had to say: 'Pamela, you know what we agreed. Do you want me to . . .?' and she would answer: 'No! Give me a minute or two . . .' The free behaviour was not in itself the therapy, nor would an imposition of sanctions without consent have been the answer, even though many children can conform in this way.

The therapy arose from the deprivation being faced and accepted; from the desire to change bad habits and accept discipline. And the discipline had ultimately to be inside oneself even if it helped for a time to have it imposed by a recognized authority figure. Indeed, it might be said that the change had already taken place before it could be outwardly acknowledged.

Another point that we had to restate for ourselves at times was that, although we had great sympathy for the children who found themselves caught up in so much confusion, and although we wished them to know that we stood alongside them and could tolerate a good deal from them while they were sorting themselves out, this did not imply any sort of approval of anti-social attitudes. A condition of going into the outside world, even for a short time, was conformity to society's requirements. Thus, the school would only make arrangements for going out, e.g. to the swimming pool, for those able to comply with usual social standards. What we gave them was the opportunity to experiment within our experiment, and one of the most valuable aspects of the experiment was that they were given time – time to look back at themselves and their situation, time to look at themselves in their current behaviour, and time for the ordinary processes of maturation to take place. We noticed the place that magic held, expressed both in the control they hoped to have over others or that they feared others had over them, and also in the way in which they hoped others would remove from them all their difficulties by giving them things or performing surgical operations. Linked to this was the ease with which some children said 'Sorry' and immediately expected that all consequences would be cancelled out. 'But I have said sorry' they would assert indignantly. When anti-social things happened it was not pretended that nobody minded them, or that no one had ever got hurt, but by refraining from retaliation we left the way open for the offender to do something about reparation – not to say sorry, but to do it, to show a feeling of concern which might later become protectiveness.

# 3
# The school in action

## DISCUSSIONS AND GROUP MEETINGS

A difficulty experienced in the early days of the small old school was getting all the children and staff to meet together so that ideas and items of information could be shared and discussed, in the absence of the formal daily religious assembly of the ordinary schools.

As most of the boys and girls admitted to the Unit could read, we decided to use one wall of the small passage-way as a notice-board. On this we put the time-table and curriculum suggestions. There was nearly always some member of staff due for leave, and notice of this was put up for everyone to see in good time. We also put up an impersonal statement about the kind of destructive behaviour which would result in withdrawal for a time of the right to attend school. These notices all needed constant renewal as they were frequently ripped down or covered with comments, as was the wall around them.

Early in 1956 another notice was added to say that it was proposed to hold a school meeting weekly on Mondays for anyone who wished to attend. The following Monday the glass screen was folded back to turn the two small class-rooms into a large meeting room. But to our surprise, when the children arrived, the boys grouped themselves on one side and the girls on the other. A topic for discussion had been suggested on the notice. Very few remarks were addressed to the Chair, but a good deal of talking together and ribald commentary took place from which the Chairman had to pick up a word here and there, repeat it, and ask if others wished to support or discuss the point of view expressed. At first the topics we provided were somewhat academic, but as the young people showed that they approved of the idea, the plan was persisted with. We put up on the wall each week notices of what we intended to discuss, and we invited written comments before the meeting (unsigned if wished). Those received were read out at the meeting. Incidents occurring during the week also came under discussion, so that a community sorting house began to emerge. Notes of three of such weekly meetings, made during or immediately after the discussions, follow:

*March 1956*

*Are punishments necessary in the ward and in the school?*
*If so, what form should they take?*
*What sort of behaviour should receive punishment?*
These questions were read out with two written answers which had been received:
(*a*) I think punishments should be given out severely, e.g. girls should go to Beech or Holly (strict security wards) if they cheek the sister.
(*b*) I think the children in this hospital should be more concerned in their lessons, e.g. maths, English, poetry. More than in boys. Boys are just a silly pastime.
*Cheek? Is that what should be punished?*
Yes.
*What sort of punishment?*
Lose ground leave.
Be sent to bed. With nothing to do. No smoking allowed.
Not sent to another ward.
Agreed. That is going too far.
Yes, that's the trouble with this hospital. There should be punishments, but they go too far.
*That is what you think should happen on the ward. Let us talk about school. Should there be punishments here?*
Yes (this was answered quite decidedly).
*What for?*
Playing up the teachers.
Going into the other class-rooms and interrupting.
Not doing what you are told.
Taking the keys.
Going into the office without permission.
*Well, if those things happen, what punishments should be given?*
Be sent back to the ward and go to bed.
Give the cane.

Yes, give the cane, then it's all over and done with.
Give lines. Give a good thrashing.
*Have any of you ever had the cane?*
Yes (here followed various boasts, and miming).
*And thrashings at home?*
Yes (various examples were given. Some excitement and much laughter).
*Did it do any good? Did you stop being troublesome?*
No. It doesn't hurt you.
You just do it again.
You don't care.
*Then it did not do you any good. Why go on having punishments?*
You have to have punishments or children would go on being bad.
They do go on, with the punishments.
*What about the teachers?*
They love to do it, give you the cane and lines and that.
It makes them feel important. Just fancy, you can give anybody the cane whenever you feel like it.
If you didn't like it, you wouldn't do it.
*Talk about this school. Do the teachers here punish you with the cane?*
No.
*With lines?*
No.
*Thrashing?*
No.
*Is punishment necessary for you then? Do you know when you are being naughty or wrong?*
Yes.
*You don't need punishment to tell you?*
No.
*Do you stop when you make up your own minds that you don't want to go on behaving badly?*

In the cross-talk that followed, it was clear that some had already found out that what we feel like inside gives us a worse punishment than other people can give us.

*13 June 1958*
The screen was opened up. There was no set formation of the tables and chairs. One of the girls put up the ironing-board and

began to iron her skirt. Two others left the meeting and went into the back room. A group of five boys went over to the other side of the meeting room and pulled the glass screen back to shut themselves off. Di kept coming in and out of the room.

The meeting began with notices of the forthcoming fortnight's closure. There were one or two voices of approval, but more wondered what they were going to do in that time.

Then we discussed the events of the afternoon before, when five or six boys had taken possession of the staff-room and had refused to come out. The idea of using the staff-room and office had been that someone seriously working might sit there away from noise and disturbance. Sid said that whoever had ordered the room first should be allowed to sit there. A teacher pointed out that since it was a staff-room which could be used by staff invitation, she queried the use of the word 'ordered'. She then asked how the meeting thought those who rushed in and refused to come out should be dealt with. Stanley was in favour of one warning being given and then sending them back to the ward. Mike objected that one warning would be all right for some, but wrong for others. He instanced Joe who had been in trouble the day before; he felt that it would be a long time before Joe could do what he was asked with only one warning.

Someone used the word 'enforced', and a teacher asked how this ought to be done. Was it by locking people out and sending others back to the ward? Robert suggested there should be a cane. Two said that they had had the cane and admitted it had not solved their problem of disobedience. What good was it? Then Mike remarked that having the cane did not stop one, it just made a boy feel vicious or resentful against the person who punished him. Sid declared that he had had a shock when he came to the hospital; he had expected to find an organized school and found instead a brawl-alley. He was asked what this had done to him. On the whole he was inclined to think he had gained more than he had lost. He thought he had lost some time, and some accumulation of factual knowledge, and had found that he was temporarily lost without the support of an organized school. Then he had been able to organize himself reasonably well and was now able to follow his own particular interests.

Mike felt that control was important and, when the staff did not give them self-control, it made him feel he could do as he liked and join in with the noisy, disturbing people. He was asked whether control imposed by the staff was self-control, or was it lack of self-control that allowed him to join in? Sid argued that control must not be too military but must be toned down to suit a particular boy or girl because, if it was stronger than they could take, they would be all the worse for it. This tied up with Mike's statement of resentment against the person who punished. Mr P inquired if they felt resentment on the ward when discipline was enforced there. Sid said he came to the school to get away from the ward. Then Mr P asked if he were retreating, and from what? Sid replied that he liked to be able to come and settle to the thing that pleased him, not to be told all the time what to do. This made Di say that on the ward there was a continual call from sister: 'Di, do this, do that,' and at school one teacher says, 'Come here,' and other teachers say, 'Go away,' etc. She got very animated and laughed as she spoke.

Frank suggested that there should be one room for workers and one for those who wanted to mess about. He said this was the point of view put forward on the ward. The charge nurse had said that those who were a nuisance in school should be sent back and he would deal with them. The girls who wanted to could go into the staff-room. The question was asked what would happen if a person not wanting to work insisted on staying in the working room? Nothing constructive was suggested. I referred back to the time when those who found it too difficult to settle came to school for only an hour, but no one wanted this to happen.

David said he felt our methods were very wrong – we should be much more strict and make people behave. The question of standards was discussed here and it was asked who should set them? David asked whether there was anything he did which he ought not to do. After a pause I suggested that he should answer the question himself. He said the staff would think he ought not to criticize the behaviour of other boys and girls. They discussed whether he should be a judge. Did he judge from his parents' standpoint? Had teachers helped to form his judgement? What would he do if he found his parents and teachers, or other adults, holding opinions contrary to each other?

Sid said we should aim at being good in order to influence other people. We should project ourselves on to them, but not too blatantly. We discussed whether we had a ready-made blueprint to which we should live. Then Sid said that there was a blueprint in Christ in the Bible. He was asked if this desire to help others should be the conscious aim of our effort to grow. Mike thought that was why the teachers were doing their job. Sid used the word selfish, and there was some exploring of what selfish meant, and whether self-growth was the same as being selfish.

## 20 *June 1958*

By now we had discarded the policy of putting up a topic for discussion which originated from the staff but relied upon suggestions which came from the boys and girls themselves. This week no topics for discussion were sent in, but several boys and one girl had said they were going to take part in the meeting. When the meeting began, three boys shut themselves off in the second part of the room (where they could nevertheless hear what was being said). Three girls went into the back room. After the meeting had started, Mike came in and sat on a table, and Yvonne came and stood just inside the door. Robert was in nearly all the time, but towards the end, when reference was made to feeling sorry for injuries which resulted accidentally from going too far, he rushed from the room. The psychologist also was present. As no specific topics were presented for the meeting it was suggested that we should consider certain things which had cropped up during the week.

*Staff break.* The mid-morning break was then discussed. I described the way in which the boys hid and wasted the time of the staff, and also how they came early at 1.30 p.m. and kicked the door, etc. The day before George had kicked a panel of wood out of the door, and all the boys had been banished for the rest of that morning. The group quickly took up this statement as an attack against George individually, but when the matter was pursued they admitted that George's incident was only part of the day's annoyance, and it was in a way accidental that it had been George and not someone else who had done the final damage. The discussion began to cover last week's ground, that there should be a warning and then punishment. I said that, in banishing the boys, we had on that occasion punished but we were now discussing it to see if we could make this unnecessary.

Should the staff have a break? Why did they want a break? Di thought they should, they needed it. Why? Sid referred to the 'schizophrenic children' who came in the first hour, and Robert talked of those who were 'up the stick' and said the staff needed a break. It seemed fairly clear that the majority thought it reasonable for the staff to have a break although there was scornful reference to tea drinking. Then Di said: 'Let them have a break and a cup of tea – it will put them into a better mood for us for the rest of the morning.'

*Destructive behaviour in general*. In introducing this point, I said we had always understood that sometimes, because they were feeling angry or dissatisfied, some people would want to tear up work they had done or to break the things they had made. Were they willing to discuss the sort of destruction we had recently had to the walls and doors, and the breaking of models, etc., belonging to other people. In the talk which followed, Muriel said she had torn up her books. Sid said that at times one felt that one must destroy what one had done. He had spoilt a picture and then had burned it, because of the rage he felt that made him froth at the mouth. Anger was given as one reason for destroying one's own things, and disappointment as another. Someone then said: 'We can destroy them if we want to, they are ours.' The staff agreed that we had always accepted that viewpoint, but wanted to know why other people's things were now being destroyed. Mike thought jealousy was a reason for destroying them. Sid said he did not think so. I asked what the group felt we should do about it? Should a line be drawn against destruction of the building? Where would we meet if we had no building? Should this behaviour be looked upon as illness, with those people who did it as too ill for the time being to come to school?

Robert said there should be punishment. Mike objected that when things were destroyed it was often done in a blind rage, and you couldn't punish someone who was in a blind rage. Were things only done in a blind rage? No. Often something quite small in itself made someone destructive because of his feelings about things which had nothing at all to do with the school. Earlier in the meeting Di had said she wanted to know why she was always picked on when Yvonne and the boys could do anything they liked. Now she said she came to school as a place where she could let herself go, because all the time she was on the ward it was: 'Di, you know how to do this,' 'Di will do that,' 'You can rely on Di,' and she was fed up with it.

The psychologist asked what they meant when they said people were 'schizophrenic' or 'up the stick', but no one was able to do more than indicate that the terms related to others, not themselves. The psychologist said she preferred just to use the word 'ill'.

Frank said he thought there should be less time for the gramophone, he got tired of hearing the same records. It was stated. that David had sung 'Tulips from Amsterdam' in his sleep, so they had to put up with it day and night too! David laughed and said that was proof that the gramophone should not be on too much. As the gramophone was only on for the children's records towards the end of the afternoon, it was agreed that those who did not like it should be free to leave; they would have to return to the ward, as normal at the end of school, and receive permission from the ward to go out elsewhere. The degree to which this freedom to leave was used would show how much the gramophone was wanted.

There had been a certain amount of minor damage due to thoughtlessness. In some cases it was only by good luck that serious injury hadn't been done. Ought we to work together to prevent these things? During the discussion that followed, someone said that we all want to be good. Mike said we did not all want to be good, we were not angels. Robert asked why were the teachers not more strict, then he left the room. Di said she knew what was wrong with her and she wanted it to stay that way because to change meant that she had got to give in, and she would never give in. She knew all she wanted to know except one thing, and there was no one she could ask. She corrected this to there was one person she could ask, but she was afraid of what the answer would be, so she was going to stay as she was.

Sid spoke of what happened when boys were sent back to the ward. They were sent to bed for three days and had nothing to do, and they stored up more hate to use against us when they came back. In the same sentence he spoke of the staff triumphing on the battlefield when someone got sent back and of the feeling of being cast out and not wanted. We tried to pursue these ideas separately. He implied that most of the time there was a tension between the children and the staff, and then came the moment of triumph for the staff, when they became the enemy. Mike said the staff were meant to have enough patience to help the children. The psychologist said Sid had referred to the staff being qualified to deal with the children – when they sent someone back to the ward they were telling him that at that point they could not cope. Did this worry him? Sid felt that it was awkward not knowing when your friend was going to be your foe. It was up to the staff to use psychology and know how to give each individual the sort of confidence he needed. He thought that he and Mike could be sent back and could think things over and be better for it. But caning would be better for a boy like Robert who would build up a hate if he were sent to bed. The psychologist said that he implied that Robert was less able to deal with his difficulties, was more ill than himself and Mike and that, in selecting caning for Robert, he was saying that being sent back to the ward was a bigger punishment than caning would be.

Mr C tried to explore with Sid whether a staff decision to return someone to the ward was always motivated by staff aggression. Sid said he thought sometimes other children were glad as well as staff if someone were sent back but he could not think of any other reason for doing so than a wish to retaliate.

At one point one of the children said that a boy would come to school with his mind made up to play up and see how far he could go, and sometimes others joined in so that staff would either have to turn them out or be turned out themselves. I asked what would happen if the staff were not strong enough and they were turned out? Sid said it was the head teacher's job to know when something had got to stop and that the staff had to be tactful and not upset people. She asked him to explain about being tactful. He replied that to have something talked about when you did not want that subject touched on was one of the things that put you into a rage and made you break out and destroy things. (The nursing tutor came in with a large group of student nurses but the discussion continued in spite of some distraction and cross-talk against the visitors.) At one point Mike said again it was the things you had on your mind before you came to school that caused the outbreak of bad behaviour. Perhaps some small incident at school was the spark, and then everything blew up.

## RELIGION

One of the matters about which we felt some concern was that of morning assembly. Working for years in other local education authority schools had accustomed the staff to the daily communal act of worship. Here, however, the times of attendance for the groups varied, and moreover, since the children often arrived in a truculent frame of mind, it seemed unsuitable to make an act of worship the first item on the programme. When the matter was discussed in the staff-room, it was felt that it should be left to each teacher to keep the matter in mind and to seize opportunities offered by groups or individuals as would be done in any other subject.

On my first day, the way I stood with a book in hand reminded one of the girls of someone in another school who had led the prayers. A boy who had come from a Rudolf Steiner school told his teacher that he had learnt a prayer in German. He repeated it, and when asked what it meant, said: 'Well, it is lifting up our hearts to the Christ Spirit.' A few days later a girl said that the ward was so noisy at night she forgot to say her prayers, so again we said them together in the class-room. Grace, a Catholic, who crossed herself when prayers were said, then announced that she did not believe in God as her family only believed in what they could prove. Others were horrified to know that there were people who did not believe in God.

Some care had to be taken in choosing prayers, as the group might contain Roman Catholics, Jews, Jehovah's Witnesses, and Protestant sects, and it never became the rule to have formal group prayers. Interest in religious topics was recurrent and showed itself in a variety of ways. Pippa, a brain-damaged girl, who had severe temper outbursts, would often come into the office, take a Bible from the shelf, settle herself down in the easy-chair, find St Matthew xi and read aloud: 'Come unto Me, all ye that are weary and heavy-laden . . .' 'I like that,' she would say, 'it makes me feel better.' Near the office door in those days a large picture map of Palestine was pasted to the wall. Near the placenames and round the border were coloured pictures of New Testament incidents. Often a boy or girl would stop by the map and say: 'I know that story, it was when . . .' The map held a fascination for Margo. She came from a convent school and her much loved elder sister was about to take her vows as a Carmelite nun. (One day when Margo was holding the dustbin lid in front of herself, one of the staff said: 'Are you hiding?' 'No,' she said, putting the lid down, 'I am not going to be a nun.') She had an explosive tic consisting of the sound of the letter 'B', and used to beat herself on the breast and jerk her arms and legs. She used to spit when annoyed or wishing to annoy, and often spat at the map. Later she took to scoring it in several places with a pair of scissors, making her explosive 'B' sound as she did so. In time she extended the 'B' to 'bugger'. She added a following 'G' sound, and then would put her hands to her mouth in horror as if trying to push the sound back. When she could speak again she would say: 'I mustn't say that.' Each time she cut the map, we mended it and finally suggested that she should say in full what the map made her feel like saying. Eventually she got round to saying: 'Bugger God.' At that time she felt she hated Him because her sister was ready to leave her for ever to go to Him. She had a delightful sense of humour and we loved having her although she often made a nuisance of herself on the ward. Gradually her breast beating, jerkiness, and explosive tic lessened. She began to write to her sister, although she found this very difficult, fearing that her interest in film stars and the latest records would appear unseemly to a nun, and she actually accompanied her parents to the ceremony at which her sister's vows were taken.

Janice, on the other hand, belonged to one of the Free Churches. She came in one day and asked if she could take a service in the office; to do this, she said, she would have to re-arrange the furniture. I agreed, and the desk was moved to one end and a number of chairs arranged in front of it in rows. On the table she placed a Bible, a prayer-book, and a hymn-book, and she provided me with a hymn-book. She asked me to sit on one of the chairs and to pretend that I was among other members of a congregation. I stipulated that the office door should remain open and that other children who came must receive attention. Janice announced that she was the clergyman and looking at me anxiously she said: 'Would you call me the Reverend?' She went outside and walked in impressively and I stood up. She chose a hymn which we sang together, and read some prayers and a passage from the Bible. Then came the sermon, a long and quite coherent commentary on the parable of the wise and foolish virgins. From time to time other children looked in and I quietly attended to them; they rolled their eyes and whispered: 'She's mad,' but made no other interruption. At the end of the sermon and another hymn the week's announcements were given, and mention was made of sick parishioners, concluding with thanks to me for help in the service. This programme frequently recurred, and she would take great pains in selecting and writing lists of prayers, hymns, and readings, but always the sermon was on the ten virgins with special emphasis on how to avoid being numbered with the foolish ones. It was not until months after her admission that I got to know of a history of sexual interference.

For most of this time Janice's behaviour had been fairly well sustained except for noisy outbursts now and again. Then she went through a very wild stage, when she was very difficult to contain in school although she loved to come. One day in this period she rushed into the office, tipped over a chair, and pushed a pile of papers off the desk. She stood laughing at the other side, then moved to a low cupboard to push the books off that. Prominent on top was a large Oxford Dictionary in a dark blue cover. She pulled herself back and said: 'Oh, that's a Bible, I mustn't touch that,' and ran out of the room. In a few seconds she was back, shouting: 'I don't care if it is a Bible' and she threw it down. Then she went to the window, opened it, and called out: 'Are you up there God? I'm going to spit on your Bible.' Turning, she made a token spit towards the book on the floor. Meanwhile, feeling that the incident was of some importance to Janice, I had closed the door and was leaning against it to prevent anyone else from coming in. Janice went back to the window and called out: 'If you don't like it, flap your wings and come down and I'll spit on you.' Then all the bluster went out of her; she closed the window and turned round, looking small and white. 'I shouldn't have said that, should I? Will He be angry with me?' I smiled and said: 'Well, you know, if I can take it, I am sure God can. What about showing Him you are sorry by helping me to put the room straight?' Janice worked quickly to restore the room to its normal state. As she went out she pressed my hand and smiled and said in an old-fashioned way that she sometimes had: 'Thank you, you are a great help to me.'

Spontaneous discussion arose at times among the children as to whether there is a God and whether as individuals they believed in him. Rufus always wore a crucifix, and when challenged by the other children he said: 'You don't believe most of the time but, when you are in trouble, you do.' Mick would carry round with him a Bible, prayer-book, and hymn-book, and arrange them carefully on his desk alongside any other books he was using. He was seldom seen to open them. Ben carried his Service book in his pocket. At one point he decided to become an active adherent of the Devil, and spent some time rewriting prayers from the book to apostrophize the Devil instead of God or Christ. When he showed these to me I concerned myself only with querying the words which he had left unaltered, such as Saviour, Redeemer, grace, salvation – were these appropriate in the new context? Finally he tore his Service book in half and gave me the pieces. Was this to have them kept safe in spite of his destructiveness? Colin became very concerned while Ben was working through this rebellion, and projected his anxiety on to me. He made a large pencil drawing of Christ on the cross, and bringing it into the office said: 'This is for you. Put it up on the wall.'

We found that a devil was often among us, sometimes cropping up in nightmarish paintings, but frequently the devil was a personal companion, haunting the consciousness of the child. Reg lived in an almost total state of fantasy and stood about with his fingers in his ears in order not to hear the terrible things that his devil told him to do. Bernadette, a highly intelligent girl who had been convent-reared, called her devil Michael; she drew pictures of him and pasted them all over the place; he looked down at us from the ceiling and up from the floor. He had slanting eyes and wore a dagger at his belt, and she would shake her hair over her face and quote him when she expressed her anti-social thoughts. Maudie, when she had come a long way out of her hallucinated state, remembered her devil and used consciously to invoke him when she wanted to regress. Lisa, who was not at all hallucinated, and who had been brought up a Methodist, blamed her behaviour on the devil who tempted her, but she was able to accept with a smile that she might sometimes listen with the other ear to the promptings of her guardian angel.

Painting and drawing, ever-present activities, provided a number of children with an opportunity to express their religious thoughts. Billie covered a large sheet of paper with splashes of paint and over the resulting confusion of colour painted in a heavy green cross, and some inches below it, a tiny brown dot which he said was himself. The cross, he said, he had put in 'just in case', and in further explanation said he thought he was not a Christian, nor did he want to believe in God, but how could one be sure? He thought it was his very best picture and he did not want to give it to the teacher. She had not asked for it and pointed out that he could do just what he wished with it. He felt he must give it to her because he wanted it to be on the wall in the office. The cross, its dominant feature, focused the eye and stimulated discussion among the other children. Once he took it down and walked out of school with it, then changed his mind and brought it back to be put up again. Later, when he had been destroying other children's work, one of them insisted that he should tear his own picture. He tried to avoid this, but an angry group hemmed him in, and slowly he climbed up and tore it across, nevertheless leaving the pieces hanging on the wall. After they had gone one of the teachers mended the picture on its back. When in answer to his query, she said briefly that perhaps one of the things the cross meant was that broken things could be made whole again, he gave a pleased nod.

Anita had a bold colourful style in her pictures, indicative, perhaps, of her energy and warmth. Her uninhibited behaviour caused a good deal of concern, of which she was aware. At times her remorse and penitence would swamp her, and then she would sit quietly and paint lovely pictures of the Madonna in traditional blue and white. Jeannette also painted the Virgin, a life-size black figure, on the window of her class-room. We found her a most depressing presence whom we could not ignore but whom we had to endure for some weeks.

Gilbert used the wall for his picture, an area of about six feet by nine feet, which took many days to complete. The centre part was a deep chasm; on the left were jagged, dark-coloured peaks, while on the right were yet higher peaks and plains shining in light. In the upper air above the chasm was a small circle decorated in geometric designs, towards which were flying from several directions dark-winged bat-like creatures. Gilbert would say little about his picture. His work on it was meticulously careful, and he would get up from his academic work at times, pick up a brush, and without a word, go to the wall to paint in a few feathers on a bat's body or to deepen a colour here or there. One day he came into the office and asked for a Bible. I gave him one and said: 'Can I help?' He hesitated, then said: 'Where does it say about the valley of death?' I handed him a prayer book and said: 'Find Psalm 23. I expect you will know it better in this version.' He went away and later we found across the top of the picture in pencilled capitals, 'Though I walk through the valley of the shadow of death I will fear no evil.' He now began to talk briefly about his picture, saying that the soul (the circle) was travelling from earth (left), to heaven (right), and assailed on the way by evil which was represented by the bats.

From then on, however, his interest in the picture declined, and the letters remained unpainted. Before long he was discharged from the hospital.

Free written work also revealed a preoccupation with religious sentiments, as in Christine's rather conventional verses:

O Lord please do forgive me
    For all the sins I've had,
Please change my life completely
    To goodness from the bad.
Please help me to in every way
    Be good and kind and helpful
From one day to the next day,
    And come when You do call.

I wish that Thou wouldst help me
    And come in my heart to stay,
And lead me to do rightly,
    Each minute, day by day.
May You help me always
    To stand up for myself
And to tell the truth always,
    And keep me to myself.

So now I come to the end of
    This prayer for forgiveness to You.
And may you never turn me off
    From doing good for You.
Please take care of all I love,
    My parents, relations, and friends,
And bring them to Thy kingdom above.
So now all this prayer ends;
Glory be to the Father above,
And glory be to the Son,
Glory be to You both I love,
And Spirit, Three in One.
                Amen.

Christmas proved to be a very difficult time each year. As the autumn term drew on into November, excitement began to rise and plans were made and often carried out for making presents for each other and members of their families. Carols were played

on the piano, record player, or guitar, and little groups gathered
to sing from carol sheets. Lucky ones received letters asking them
to go home for the holiday. But as the time drew nearer, early
December, mid-December, so the tension grew. Christmas is
essentially a family time. Those who had no families found their
loneliness accentuated at this season; those who had families
idealized the situation until the time came for the reunion, when
they realized even more forcibly that their homes were not
havens of peace and joy with loved ones. Some even accepted
with relief the doctor's recommendation that they were not well
enough to go home, although they shouted vociferously against
the decision in order to cover the emptiness. More than one child
could be heard, any year, saying bitterly that he hated Christmas.

One Christmas soon after I arrived at the school, we decided
to hold a Christmas service. Great interest had been shown in
practising carols, three girls had asked if they might be among the
readers, and preparations had gone well. The large hall of the
hospital (there was no chapel) had been put at our disposal, and
on the day we went off to hold our service. Then it was we found
how hopeful our travelling had been compared with our arrival.
Various doors led into and from the hall, and we spent much
time in retrieving children who went in by one and straight out
by another, the three readers among them. At last we got started,
but the readers were either too frightened or too self-conscious
to do their part; one interrupted her reading and threatened to
'bash' someone who was watching her if he did not turn his gaze
away, and another interpolated unseemly words into the text.
For a long time after that we let our singing and listening to
Christmas music be spontaneous.

More recently, under the compelling enthusiasm of a member of
the staff, a talented Welshman, a Nativity Play was staged in one
of our class-rooms. The play consisted largely of a set of tableaux
(with some movement) introduced by and interspersed with carols
and readings. The casting was carefully done, and we were
fortunate to have on the staff a British Guianaian with a good
voice who took the part of one of the kings. A good deal of
thought went into the making of the props and the dresses were
beautiful, for we had spent quite a bit on acquiring some lovely
pieces of material. The author/producer went to much trouble to
rig up curtain poles and runners and to train a stage manager and
the interest and enthusiasm of the staff was shared by the children.

By unanimous choice Millie was selected as Mary. Millie was one of those children who refused to talk but she had a gentle, smiling expression and looked very sweet sitting by the crib. There was no baby within the crib, only a light, as we knew from experience that certain children might subject the substitute object to many indignities. We had been particularly pleased at the interest shown by one boy who had agreed to be the innkeeper. Just before the performance, however, when other members of the Unit staff, doctors, psychologists and nurses came in, he became too frightened to do more than stand at the side of the stage, and another boy shook so badly that he had to be held for a time. Afterwards coloured transparencies of the show gave great pleasure, and the innkeeper had a fantasy in which he saw himself producing the entire play the following year.

Arrangements for religious observance were made by the hospital authorities in conjunction with ministers of various denominations. Services were held on Sundays and certain week-days. Val always came late to school on Wednesday mornings because she had been to the mid-week celebration of Holy Communion. For years there was no full-time chaplain, but an Anglican clergyman visited each of the juvenile wards once a week to take a Bible class. Since he and other clergy used to come into school now and again unannounced, as seems to be the way in hospital, and with an extraordinary disregard for any other adult whom they might encounter, there was little opportunity for talking over common problems. Only the infrequent visits of the Free Church minister and the Jewish Rabbi were marked by warmth and courtesy. The Anglican clergyman considered all the children to be feeble-minded, and advocated keeping their hands constantly employed.

Although the formal act of worship was not included in the school programme, a fair amount of material was available for religious instruction as a subject, with pictures and verses to colour, quizzes on Bible material, models to make, and books to read. Often a Bible character or incident was included in the weekly drama session, but the real spiritual work was probably done in individual contacts, when outbursts of anger, hatred, or bitterness provided an opportunity to consider the alternative possibilities of forgiving and loving.

## SEX

In this age group, without any outside stimulation, interest in sex was dominant. Some made great attempts to conceal their interest, some resented their ignorance, and others seemed to have no time for any other ideas and flaunted their preoccupation with sex in their speech. Some girls regarded their changing appearance with fear and tried to hide it, walking with round shoulders and sitting with arms folded to conceal their growth. Others hailed their bodily changes with joy as a sign that the bondage of childhood was ending and that they were now 'grown-up'.

At one time a good deal of anxiety was aroused on the ward if it were known that a boy had homosexual leanings; homosexual activities were punished by the staff and by the other boys in whom great guilt and much righteous indignation were aroused. The other boys tended to continue the attack in school and to make known to the girls why they were ganging up against a particular boy. Masturbation was also a reason for punishment and ostracism. Once there were full-time ward doctors, these things were dealt with differently. In school we neither criticized nor condoned. We wanted them to see that they had adopted these interests in an attempt to remain unconscious of other and worse problems, and this was one of the reasons why hospital treatment was necessary. At the same time, as far as possible, we eliminated dark corners and empty rooms that made it easier to give in to temptation.

Most of the boys who showed homosexual tendencies went on to become heterosexual and, in time, their interest in and friendship for girls predominated. Others could discuss the problem intellectually and dispassionately (unlike those innocent and unwilling victims of sexual assaults who showed great anxiety and distress) and refused to relinquish an activity which they found satisfying. One such was Dermot who voluntarily wrote his life story in which he told how, as an only son, he was a frequent witness of quarrels between his parents which ended several times in his mother leaving home. He and his parents moved from place to place, and each time Dermot hoped in vain that the new place would give them happiness. Now he was dressing up as a girl and going out. He was an attractive-looking, dark-haired boy, who accepted petting from strangers. Attempts had been made through a local clinic and, later, a day hospital to help him to accept a male rôle. He was involved in a court case, and seemed to have acquired from it a feeling of power, and on subsequent occasions he accepted relationships with men and then informed against his companions. For a while when he was with us he teamed up with Vi. She was a girl, who, like himself, had difficulty in accepting her sexual identity; she longed to be a boy, wore her hair short and straight, dressed in front-zipping jeans and sweaters, was athletic and followed boys' pursuits. Their partnership enabled them to look as though they were following a heterosexual pattern but, in fact, they made no demands on each other. The other children were not fooled by their alliance and, in the end, they did not even try to keep up the pretence of being interested in each other. Finally, Dermot decided to go home and, if he could not endure the parental wrangling, to move into a hostel.

One of the difficulties we had to contend with was the facile way in which emotionally loaded words were misused by other grown-ups in discussing personalities with the children. 'Schizophrenic' and 'M.D.' were used inaccurately and tauntingly and 'Lesbian' and 'Homo' were thrown at any child who showed any preferences for the company of one of his (or her) own sex.

For the main periods of the day the class groupings in the school were singled sexed. This had largely been decided upon by an earlier stream of children, who, when the classes had been mixed, found that owing to the accident of discharge dates one girl might remain alone among a group of boys, or vice versa. However, boys and girls could meet on common ground in the office and in the communal activities of drama and for the last half hour of the day with the gramophone. Moreover, any boy or girl, with the consent of the two teachers concerned, could work for a time in another group room.

Sometimes a very strong attachment would spring up between a boy and a girl so that for a time they could hardly tolerate separation. The youngsters concerned were usually intelligent and sensitive who from an early age had been faced with personal loneliness and lack of maternal support. These young people would make the quite intense attachment to each other that is sometimes seen in an infants' school when two little children love each other. Unfortunately their position was complicated, because they were not in fact little children and suspicion and hostility would be aroused against them, arising from anxiety, especially as the place was not sufficiently well staffed for unobtrusive surveillance to be maintained.

These over-intensive types were exceptional. Most boys and girls showed a normal interest in sexual matters but with some there was too much inhibition and with others too little. Jean would dance round with her skirts lifted regardless of time or company, and Charles would put on a poker-face if the slightest and most ordinary reference were made to bodily or toilet matters. Sex and excretion were confused, and talk of both was indulged in often, in attempts both to shock and also to test whether an adult might safely be asked some more serious question. The attitude of the school staff in general was not to be shocked but, at the same time, to keep a reasonable balance as to what was permitted when, and, indeed, to whom. Active expression by the inhibited was to be encouraged, and sometimes to tolerate an exhibitionist was a means of giving confidence to the over-frightened. Often, we realized too, some showed an excessive interest as a way of concealing fear.

Straightforward factual answers were given to questions on intercourse and birth. We did not object to scrap-books of bathing beauties, and pin-ups were allowed on the walls. Sketches of a nude woman were sometimes thrust upon one of the women teachers, or fixed with her name attached, with a great display of daring, on the wall of the office, to be removed usually by some child who could not tolerate them. It would be 'reflected back' to both types of children 'you want to think about this', 'you do not like to think about this,' which usually led to further comment and discussion, and in any case served to indicate that such thoughts were not going to be punished as 'wicked' or 'dirty'.

The sexual precocity of some of the boys and girls was a source of worry to the staff and, as opportunity offered, or was made, straight talks were given individually on the results of uncontrolled and promiscuous behaviour. I would use my position as school mother to speak in lieu of their own mother. They might toss their heads and say: 'Thank God you are not my mother,' or say that they knew how to take care of themselves, or 'Cheek, I am not like that.' But, in fact, they were usually glad that we showed concern and dealt openly with a situation which at times threatened to get beyond them. It did get beyond a few of them. Joyce, a green-eyed merry youngster, was both irresistible and unresisting; even Ray, a tall self-contained boy who had no eyes for a girl until Joyce came, was at her feet. But Joyce was a wanderer who, for the sheer joy of freedom, absconded from time to time, accepting lifts from car or lorry drivers and bringing herself back when the fling was over. She came one morning to ask how a girl would know if she were pregnant. A very worried little girl was talking, her factual knowledge and her worldly-wiseness had not restrained her sexual propensities any more than lack of such knowledge makes for innocence and self-restraint. Actually, Joyce's pregnancy proved a turning point in her situation. Her child was not the first illegitimate one in her family, and her parents received her as an adult when she returned home.

Some of the sex interest was entirely at a fantasy level; a girl would claim that she had had intercourse and that her baby had been removed, and more than one boy described himself as the supporting husband and father of a family of several children. Since such strong fantasies rendered ordinary human contacts unnecessary, it was a step towards health when a child of this sort began to make ordinary friendships. Mavis was a pretty, potentially intelligent girl whose illness had distorted her looks and her behaviour. She attended the school for a long time and received sustained individual therapy from the psychologist at a time when little intensive help of this kind was being offered in the Unit. For months she was an outcast among the other girls, who classed her among those they cruelly called 'the dossy ones' and, as the boys took their cues from the girls, it was difficult for her to achieve her desire to belong. Among the boys was tall, quiet Paul, who, it appeared later, was genuinely subnormal in intelligence and unable to compete at the same speed as the others, but whose behaviour was socially acceptable. Mavis used Paul to acquire the prestige enjoyed by girls who could secure a boy friend. He was bewildered by her attentions, but was amenable and quite safe for her. She was artistic, and now that she was getting better, able to take the initiative. Along with the other girls she designed and painted a valentine, and gave hers to Paul; she persuaded him to venture on to the dance floor and arranged that he should escort her to and from the ward and school. The other children became interested in this friendship and made room for Paul and Mavis to be included in their company. Both had been in a sense outsiders; now they had acquired status which Mavis retained after Paul's discharge.

Two girls, Pat and Jane, both had difficulties in making an acceptable relationship and their ardour frightened the boys into openly beating them off. Pat was longing to return home and, as her severe temper outbursts had subsided, her parents were ready to have her, but how would she survive in the general community if she continued to rush at men and boys to molest them sexually? The doctor did not appear to realize the intensity of this urge because, for the short periods of their interviews, she was on her best behaviour. We had, therefore, to help her to make best behaviour ordinary behaviour. A very studious boy, whose intellectual and artistic ability earned him great respect from the other youngsters, struck up a platonic friendship with her. She was not above average intelligence but she was able to share his interest in classical music. She found that it was possible for her to sit with a boy and walk and talk with him without being sexually stimulated. He knew of her difficulty and encouraged her to control it. Again, their friendship, as they were of opposite sexes, gave them status in the adolescent society, but its great value to Pat was that it gave her time to grow out of what was possibly her own fear of sexual attack. Jane, too, was over-exuberant in her desire to have a boy friend, and would fling herself on the boys and kiss them and embarrass them by her verbal obscenities, as well as by the way she threw up her skirts. For her, too, it was probably fear which caused this behaviour, for she would scream, run, look back in the hope of being chased, and scream again if she were. One of the older members of the staff showed her great courtesy, e.g. offering her his arm in the walk down the corridor, partnering her sometimes in a waltz, and speaking to her always as if she were a grande dame. She blossomed under this treatment and the boys were able to see that, if they were gentle with her, she tangled less with them. After months with us she was able to reveal that a man had involved her in a sexual relationship while she was still at the primary school.

Such incidents to little girls seemed to result in one of two differing lines of behaviour, creating in the child either an excited fear (or a fearful excitement), as a result of which she behaved as Jane did, or a feeling of great degradation, in which the girl saw herself as damaged and worthless and felt certain that what had happened to her was because of her own intrinsic badness. Her attitude, therefore, became one of complete hopelessness and inertia, or of challenge through hostile behaviour, often actually accompanied by the words: 'You see how bad I am, no one can like me.' This was Lily's pattern, and again it took several months of tolerating extremely difficult behaviour before she was able to reveal that her foster father used to have intercourse with her in a small shed in the garden. Even when she had brought herself to the point of telling me this, she could not face me. She sat in a swing-chair, turned herself to the wall, and bade me stand behind her where she could not see my face. After some days I persuaded her to go with me to tell this to the doctor, but in his presence Lily was again so overcome with shame that she could only nod dumbly when I said 'Shall I tell him?' The doctor was very gentle and understanding with her and managed to put her at her ease. It was the first of many talks that she had with him and, ultimately, Lily was able to take her place satisfactorily in a girls' boarding school.

During the years in which the Unit was working there was a noticeable change in the attitude of the girls themselves towards showing their feelings about sex. At the beginning they tried to keep their feelings hidden and felt guilty when, in spite of themselves, their interest broke through in dreams and day-dreams, in their art, in what they wrote, or said. Much of their behaviour was furtive, with embarrassed laughter. Later they were more open, not necessarily with more sincerity or very deep feelings, for they wanted the status of having a boy friend and as one friend was cast off another was taken on as easily as a change of hairstyle. They usually preserved the basic idea of modesty, however, and upheld morality quite earnestly. Nevertheless, with a few there was a hardness, almost a brazenness, when they boasted of sexual experience and know-how. As with Jean, much of this was bravado, a measure of their fear and the only way of defence they knew. Candy was a lovely girl who, in spite of her family background, had high personal standards. All the boys and indeed some of the male nurses wanted her favour. Young as she was, she used every weapon in her armoury and enjoyed her supremacy. At times, however, it exhausted her and she would beg to come and sit in the office where she could be quiet and alone, at ease with her lessons, free from emotional strain. After a week-end away, she came in and sat; after a while, in a low tone, she said: 'I'm not a virgin any longer.' I responded to what I felt was her deep disappointment in herself. It was a sad moment, but one in which she grew up. She was greatly helped throughout by a boy

who also had great personal charm, and who, moveover, was a
fighter whom the other boys respected. He was not truly established as heterosexual but, for status value, usually took a girl
around. He seemed to understand the predicament which Candy
sometimes found herself in, and would become her escort and
defender whenever she needed a respite from her other too
fervent admirers. At times two boys would fight over one girl,
and a girl would sometimes secure her ascendancy over other
girls by urging her boy friend to fight their boy friends. Yet there
was much gentleness and loving understanding among these
young people as well as the aggression and hostility that were
more easily noticed because of the accompanying noise.

Now and again an older boy's interest in a girl would provide
the necessary stimulus for him to face up to reality. When he
claimed that he was considering marriage we would ask: 'Where
are you going to live? Who will pay the rent? What will you live
on? When you have a child, who will look after it?' and so on,
and these questions and their answers did, indeed, lead some of
them on to consider a more adult approach to life and its
responsibilities.

Mostly, however, interest in sex took its place as one among
many other interests and the children found socially acceptable
ways of channelling increased awareness of each other: walking
and talking together, engaging together in artistic and intellectual
pursuits, dancing, listening together to music, sharing their
thoughts with a look or touch of the hand, making things for
each other and doing small services for one another. A girl would
wash and iron her boy friend's shirt, he would mend her broken
bracelet or locket, they would cook for each other and choose
records which conveyed what they wanted to say to each other.

Play activities revealed not only an interest in sex as such, but
an interest in birth and death, in physical aggression between the
sexes, in sibling reactions, and in the fear of parents, particularly,
perhaps, of the mother or woman. Among small children the
game of 'Mothers and Fathers' is ageless. Among these older
children there was a reversion to these games of infancy with
later experience added. A boy would dress up as a pregnant
woman with a bundle pushed in among his clothes to represent
the baby. Sometimes this was afterwards taken out and gently
dandled; sometimes it was allowed to fall heavily to the ground
to be subsequently kicked about. Damp sand in the sand tray

was moulded into a woman's torso and cut into; clay figures were modelled, sometimes lifelike; others were abstract, phallic and bowl-like, which other children would interpret. Among newcomers to the Unit, anxious glances would then be cast at the staff, but when the only comment from a teacher was a technical one, relaxation would lead to confidence which enabled the teacher to be treated in due course as a friend who might be able to help.

# 4
# Therapeutic education

It hardly needs saying that in our school, because it was a 'special' school and, still more, because it was a hospital special school, a normal secondary school programme would not do. For one thing, the length of time we had for working with any child was usually short and always unpredictable. Occasionally, it is true, our wishes prevailed and we were permitted to continue with a child but, for the most part, patients were discharged from the hospital and left our school when the doctors thought they ought to leave. It would have been futile to have planned a course lasting for several years or even for one year. Secondly, although the school was small, the range of ages was wide; the range of mental ages was wider still, and attainments varied most of all. At one end of the scale were a few children capable of succeeding in G.C.E. or even University entrance examinations; at the other quite a number who had never learnt to read or to make the most elementary arithmetical calculation. Some seemed never to have used pen, pencil, or paintbrush. Of these, some saw that they had a disability and were keen to overcome it before they went to work but others had long since abandoned hope and, when they first came, could not settle to any activity, academic or practical.

Many could not concentrate or were convinced that they could not, some were intolerably anxious, some restless or aggressive. For such as these we had to make school a place where they could be helped to become accessible to therapy. It was more important to restore their confidence than to give education. First, they needed to experience the relationships of a good home and then, to be helped to grow up emotionally so that, sooner or later, they would be able to make relationships with people who

demanded more of them than we did. For the child to gain
confidence, to acquire some insight into his own inner world,
and learn to control his feelings, mere change of environment was
not enough. He had to be given opportunities to re-experience
traumatic events of the past, to bring his fantasies into the open;
in short, he had to be allowed to regress. As far as was consistent
with safety, the school and school equipment were the children's
to use as they wished. Group discussions were held in which they
could listen to one another talking of their problems; we had to
provide remedial teaching to help them overcome feelings of
inferiority, and we had to show appreciation of their work,
however inadequate from an adult's standpoint it might be. Each
child had to be given opportunities to shine, so that together the
teachers and children should make a milieu in which the children
felt themselves accepted because they were acceptable people.
Gradually their anxieties lessened or became bearable. When the
school started, none of this sort of work was being done on the
wards where regression and aggression were repressed, sometimes with severity. Recently this work has been done more
specifically by doctors and lay therapists, but for some years,
more was done within the school than outside it.

IMAGINATION, RECREATION, PLAY, AND GAMES

*Art*

When a disturbed child was faced with the problem of filling in
a period of time and was too distracted to make a consciously
controlled effort in the use of words and figures, something more
suitable had to be provided. Accordingly, we provided materials
which offered outlets ranging from mere fiddling between the
fingers to the creation of beautiful things which gave pleasure to
the maker and the beholder. Large sheets of paper of various
sorts were available at all times. Powder paint in a wide range of
colours was put out dry in bun-tins. Boxes of water-colours were
bought from time to time, and fabric printing colours, and some
of the children brought in their own oil-paints.

Techniques in painting varied a great deal; some of the children
liked to stand before a large surface and paint on the walls. In
addition to the wall picture of the soul's journey already described,
we had a scene of prehistoric animals among jungle foliage, a
huge under-water scene of fishes and plants, a fir-clad island, a

street scene with buses, and so on. Others painted on paper but appropriated a section of wall for displaying their work only. Certain types of picture occurred again and again, not only in the work of a particular child, but in the accumulated work of the school over a long period of time. These included witches, devils, monsters, graveyards, gibbets, crosses, heads of all kinds from distorted masks to idealized 'pretty' faces, and attempts at portrait painting and sketching from an actual sitter. Landscapes without figures occurred frequently, often with a fence cutting the picture in half. Houses were innumerable, mostly the front elevation only without any attempt at perspective, sometimes with no door, closed windows, strongly fenced-in garden. In the work of an individual child this might change in the course of time to a flower decked garden and a gay house with smoke from its chimneys and people at the windows and door. When house pictures were drawn, the child might be asked: 'Whose house is it? Who lives there?' and then be invited to tell what the person liked and did, so that a word story was built up around it. Or another piece of paper would be quickly provided, and another, and another, with the invitation: 'Now do the next bit of the story . . . and the next . . .'

A few of the pictures dealt in caricature fashion with hospital life with perhaps a nurse with a hypodermic syringe or a be-gowned teacher and cane. Battle scenes were frequent and included air attacks on ships, modern aerial forces bombing men with bows and arrows near a mediaeval castle, hand-to-hand fights between cowboys and Indians, outer space creatures attacking humans, and explosions all over the place. Some of them were described as bad dreams, some had named protagonists. Usually one's own side was backed to win, but in some pictures the odds against it were obviously overwhelming.

Several children preferred the quick results of making charcoal sketches, others worked in pencil or pen, making meticulous drawings in the greatest detail, every brick, every twig or blade of grass, every hair added with painful concentration. Some pictures were dark and heavy with thickly applied paint without any saving gleam of light; sometimes a picture that started gaily enough would be obliterated with great streaks of black painted over it. Others would be full of bright sketches in a jumble of ideas placed all over the paper, with curling lines in and around them and letters or words occurring among them.

Heather's pictures for a long time were scenic; a background mountain divided from the pasture in the foreground by a strong fence running right across the picture in which no people or animals were featured. Was the fence shutting her out or keeping her in? Was there an unseen figure, not yet in the picture who would intrude into the pasture or storm the mountain? Magda's pictures often contained the Devil; was he the devil within her or did he personify something or someone in her environment, present or past, who threatened and frightened her? Every one of Bob's pictures contained something horrific – a car opening up its bonnet mouth to swallow a pedestrian, a drunken man throwing a child into flames, stabbings, and hangings. Was it his own aggression finding an acceptable way out, or his terror at the violence which he felt was inherent in every situation impinging on him, or both? The teachers would ask a child to tell the story of his picture, but often he was inarticulate; he had spoken in the painting itself and other language was not available for describing his fantasies and fears. Sometimes another child, unasked, would come out with an interpretation. Then, either the artist would accept the interpretation with a knowing smile, or with fierce anger he would cry: 'It is my picture, he is not to talk about it.'

A good deal of the endless production was, however, extremely immature, and looked like the work of pre-school children although it had been executed with care and pleasure. Here it was the satisfaction of the child which had to be noted, not the result-ant piece of work, but any work had to be given a place on the wall as graciously as an effort with more obvious artistry. Terry, a fourteen-year-old from an approved school, brought into the office one day a roughly torn out paper shape daubed over in bright colours and still dripping wet. He had it flat across his hands, and exhibited it without a word, his face grave. I looked at it for a while, then nodded and said: 'Did you do this?' He said 'Yes,' and his face relaxed. I asked: 'And you are pleased with it?' Again he said 'Yes,' then added that he would like me to have it. When it had dried, we mounted it on a piece of card, to retain its shape, and hung it on the wall. Some days later he brought in a small model garage made very roughly from balsa wood. He then said he would paint it. When this was done, not very skilfully, he said with the greatest pleasure that these were the first two things he had ever done completely by himself. The rough immaturity of these products suggested that they were in

truth made, not by the fourteen-year-old boy, but by the three-
or four-year-old within him. Another boy in the hospital school,
having made a beautiful clay head which was later bronzed over,
repudiated it although he admired it, because its making had been
so controlled and modified throughout by his teacher that in the
boy's view it was the teacher's work, not his. Some of the
children, however, might be critically aware of their own inability
at a certain point to achieve what they had in mind and ask the
teacher to show them how to do it, or even to do a bit for them.
Each would attribute to the other some of the success achieved
and this helped establish a good child–teacher relationship.
There were, too, the lazy ones (or the too much damaged ones?),
who would willingly have been carried entirely by the teacher,
and from whom the teacher had to withdraw bit by bit so that
they should learn to rely upon their own efforts.

Not all the children made an instant response to the paper,
paint, chalk, etc., provided, and often the negative reply, 'I'm
no good at art' was heard. When they were sure that their work
would not be criticized, and that they could screw up what they
had done without even having to show it to anyone if they so
wished, they became bold enough to try and sometimes aston-
ished themselves with the results. A noisy tiresome child would
often become quiet when absorbed in colouring a picture printed
in outline, or painting a plaster of Paris or clay model, and would
at the same time listen to a story being read or join in a topic that
was being discussed.

Clay was one of those materials that was used spontaneously a
great deal when it was in vogue to do so and completely ignored
at other times. It would be offered to a child who had aggressive
hands, and certain preparatory rituals were gone through to
emphasize that it was a privilege, and to minimize the horse-play
which was at times suggested by it. So, a table or part of the
window bench would be assigned to the clay worker. He would
roll up his sleeves and have a large rubber apron tied round him,
but as the purpose of giving the clay was to channel off some
of the aggression, banging and noisy manipulation had to be
expected. Clay would be offered also to the children who showed
marked lack of aggression in the hope that transforming the
material with punches and pinches into an attractive object, would
remove some of the fear that aggression must be completely
destructive. Very often the clay was just played with, rolled

between the hands, and enjoyed simply because of its malleability. Free association with bodily functions was often made and was communicated to other children, sometimes with embarrassment, sometimes with complete naturalness.

Clay heads, animals, birds, people in various poses, fruit, leaves, bowls, ashtrays, and abstract shapes were modelled. We had no kiln, but the models were painted and varnished and lasted long enough. Some met with a violent end; as often at the hands of their maker as from another aggressor. Other pieces made lovingly, and as lovingly preserved, were packed up and taken as presents to people at home.

## Crafts

A number of crafts had a fairly constant place in the children's esteem; others, such as weaving, appealed only to one here and there. The making of plaster of Paris models from rubber moulds, although it might be condemned at first glance as non-creative, was a useful introduction for the hyper-active child who had to achieve something quickly. Its virtues were that it needed no skill and gave quick success. This success was usually enough to ensure that the child would sit down to paint and varnish the model. By the time that a series of plaster models had been made the child was ready to make some other sort of model, in clay, papier-mâché, or wood.

Boys who wished to do woodwork seriously and were sufficiently controlled to be allowed to use sharp tools went, on the doctor's recommendation, twice a week to the hospital adult woodwork centre and made some very nice things there. A number who tried it found that they could not accept the discipline and gave up. Each of the boys' rooms in the school had a woodwork bench and some tools, and in the winter things like sledges and go-carts were knocked together out of solid timber, but most of the model-making done was in balsa wood, using knives and a fret-saw machine. Aeroplanes, boats, and kites were the favourite objects. All sorts of items used in drama were made, and some of the boys made intricately built-up models of farms, villages, goods yards, bridges, etc. Jim made little working models of automatic machines, his favourite being one that for a three-penny bit delivered a sixpence.

The school also possessed a small printing press which was used for a time to print Christmas cards and to head sheets of notepaper with the school address (an incentive to get a few letters written!), but during one of the periodic break-ins to the cupboards, the type got badly mixed and much of it was lost. A printing set of rubber letters on wooden blocks was used a great deal by some children, and an old typewriter received a lot of use; this was in addition to the one kept for serious typing practice in conjunction with a set of records.

Every year the hospital organized a fancy dress dance and, although clothes could be borrowed from a central store, accessories were made in school, e.g. a top hat for Mad Hatter was made from cardboard covered with paper and painted. Cardboard hat-making became a major industry at times, Foreign Legion styles with cloth attached and white toppers were the favourites, some of the girls looking extremely attractive in the latter.

In the girls' rooms two sewing-machines were in constant use. Boys were allowed to use them but only under the strictest supervision for they seemed to whistle screws out of vital places. The school was seldom without at least one boy who was a menace where screws were concerned, removing them so unobtrusively that no one knew of his activity until a lock fell to pieces or small attachments vanished. The girls used the machines for making frocks, skirts, blouses, underwear, nightwear, aprons, and felt toys. Some embroidery was done and some knitting. The views of the girls were sought in the buying of pretty cotton materials. To make and wear new clothes in popular styles had a very helpful effect on their morale. They were also helped to mend and alter their clothes, to wash and iron them, and to keep pleats pressed in. Boys sometimes made shirts with a good deal of help, but they liked to use the sewing-machines to make boat sails, banners, bags, aprons for their mothers, and clothes for puppets. Before jeans became almost an adolescent uniform, it was the practice for the boys to 'peg' their trousers, machining in a leg seam to make them so narrow that it was remarkable that they could get into them at all. Constant help was sought by the boys in patching and putting back zip-fastenings and in other minor repairs such as replacing buttons, darning jerseys, and mending torn pockets.

Cooking sessions were among the most popular. If too scared at first to be ambitious with cake or pastry, the children found few problems in toasting bread, frying an egg, or making toffee. Pastry-making or dough mixing proved a good substitute for messing about with clay, and was more acceptable than clay would have been to the child who feared to see dirty hands. Moreover, the cooking materials could be eaten – either before or after cooking – and became the sole property of the maker, to be consumed then and there, or to be taken away, or cut up and shared, or to be donated completely as a present. Sometimes the recipe had been the child's own invention. Often it proved to be a reason for his consenting to read; an occasion for using the knowledge he had acquired of quantities and times; or it simply gave proof to the child that it was within his or her scope to settle to an activity with pleasurable results. Also it brought to mind memories of home and mother.

Birthdays were acknowledged by an increased issue of ingredients so that a fruit-cake could be made which was subsequently iced and decorated. The girls sometimes pooled all their allowances and made a party spread for the birthday child. Every year cakes of various kinds were baked and given to the cake-stall at the hospital's fête. One year several of the children won prizes for their cooking, but we avoided the idea of competition in the school, preferring that each should try and better his own standard without detriment to the position of someone else. No charge was made for the ingredients unless it was found that a too enterprising youngster was organizing outside sales.

Present-making, based on whichever activity appealed most to the child concerned, went on all through the year, reaching its highest peaks at Christmas and Easter, but birthdays, Mothers' Day, and special holiday seasons all called for at least one gift to be prepared. Cards, too, were designed and painted for all sorts of occasions. Some children who went home each week-end seemed unable to do so unless they went gift in hand to mark, perhaps to buy, their re-entry into the home circle.

Food was altogether a most important item, even apart from the cooking. It was, of course, provided in abundance on the wards, yet again and again a child would come and say: 'I am starving, can you give me something?' or 'I'm hungry, feed me' or would stand wordless wtih mouth opening and shutting like a baby bird. The demand was always responded to; the 'something' they were given was a sweet, or two lumps of sugar, or a slice of bread to be toasted. Two scraps of paper which have survived read: 'A nourishment capsule, please' and 'Please make me a bag of toffee.' When a firm relationship was known to exist, I would sometimes say: 'Food is to create energy – now go and do some work for me,' or 'You go and use up your energy on some work and I will replace it for you with some sugar.' A child who persistently clamoured for sweets or sugar or bread and remained generally unco-operative might at length be faced with the words: 'Now you give me a sweet.' When he replied that he had no sweet to give, he would be met again with the demand: 'But I want one. Get me one. I give you one when you ask me. Now you give me one.' After some perturbation this often resulted in the child saying that, when he next had some, he would give me one. This promise was usually kept and would be referred to with a bright smile several times: 'I gave you one of my sweets, didn't I? I said I would and I did. Did you like it?' and more than once it proved to be the beginning of the child's being able to give things, pieces of work, and little services, which were appreciatively accepted by others in the community

Basketry suited those children who liked something that grew quickly into a useful article. It had an additional value in that it required a certain amount of preparation to which they had to attend themselves; in getting the cane soaked and the uprights cut; and the end products could differ in size, shape, and ultimate colour, for often they were painted. A special gift to take home might be a basket filled with home-made toffee or a holder containing a small flowering plant.

## *Music and dancing*

The school was very fortunate for some years in having on the staff two people who were themselves competent musicians and who could inspire in the children an interest in listening and in attempting to master the skill of performing on an instrument. Mr D played the guitar and taught it and in school willingly gave of his expert knowledge to a number of boys and girls who wanted to learn to play it. At one time the school owned three guitars, and several youngsters brought in their own instruments; one even made his own guitar in his weekly session at the adult woodwork centre. The first wish of those anxious to play was to accompany a pop song and for this a few chords would suffice, doubtless they saw themselves rising to heights of fame and fortune as certain teenage idols had done. When they found out that application and energy and at least some know-how were as necessary for success in this field as in others, some were willing to give enough time and trouble to make appreciable progress. Besides earning for them almost immediately the admiring interest of their fellows, the guitar seemed of itself to provide them with companionship, they embraced it, they watched it, they listened to it, and they communicated through it; at times they sang with it or enabled others to do so. Moreover, it gave them for a time the right to one teacher's complete attention, and it secured for them the privilege of going by themselves into a room to practise.

Learning to play the piano also conferred these privileges and gave both private and public satisfaction. One boy, who had consistently used his intelligence to avoid co-operation with teachers in reading and number, accepted tuition at the piano. In this new area, not marked by previous failure, he not only made progress himself but passed on his newly acquired skill to another boy. Pianos were a great thing in the school. Every room had one of a sort, which had, before starting its life with us, earned an honourable discharge in another school or a private home. With us it had to stand up to very fierce treatment as a percussion instrument and to provide outlet for noisy aggression. Unfortunately it was difficult to separate its usefulness as a musical instrument from the fascination it had for the boy who liked to explore its inside working. For a time we had a sort of graveyard of old pianos, as we found it most difficult to dispose of what was left by our strippers, until one boy undertook to reconstruct a usable instrument out of the pieces. He worked patiently for weeks, his work being watched with great interest by others, who were allowed to help at times. The reconstructed instrument which finally resulted from his labour was gratefully received by a group teacher in exchange for the less good one in her room. For the benefit of those who wanted a musical instrument one piano was kept throughout in good condition and tuned at frequent intervals.

Other instruments which served the double purpose of standing up to a banging and producing some satisfying sounds and rhythms were drums, xylophone, cymbals, and tubular bells. Our aim that these should be used by a group in disciplined work was sometimes achieved, but often a child would use one on his own, concentrating for a long time on getting a desired result. We had to be careful when, and by whom, the drums were played. The sustained reverberating thythm which gave the greatest satisfaction to the performer sometimes worked other children up into a frenzy, and there were times when the staff could not stand it either. At a lighter level, the drum often became a rallying point for a group of boys (not by any means only the younger ones), who would follow the drummer with a hastily contrived banner or flag carried aloft in front of them, up and down the corridor, in and out of rooms, and round the building, with a zest that was complete in itself. They did no damage on their way though occasionally trouble arose not from those absorbed in the activity, but from joiners in, who could be relied on to make a mischievous contribution.

A later acquisition was a small zither with an ingenious setting out of the notes of well-known tunes by means of which the most untutored could produce a recognizable tune. One boy who completely lacked concentration in other directions spent a long time successfully transposing the zither music to the piano. From time to time, too, the school owned a number of harmonicas, which some boys played very skilfully but, as they were easily pocketable, some were lost for a season and some altogether. One of the older boys who was transferred to another psychiatric hospital wrote to us to ask if he might borrow a harmonica as it had given him such pleasure. We sent him one to keep, wondering whether apart from his success in playing he also needed the oral activity which this instrument supplied.

Several times a number of boys formed themselves by their own initiative into a music-making group. One such group acquired a tea-chest and wash-board, and formed a skiffle group. They begged to take these 'instruments' to the ward, and since they had little there to occupy them and the charge nurse favoured the suggestion, we thought it right to agree, although the activity was thereby lost to the school. One of the difficulties in continuity of interest in these groups was the frequency of admissions and discharges and, as the boys most able to take the initiative were usually those who were recovering, it was often the leader of the group who was discharged. Without him, the group tended to break down.

Another spontaneous group formed itself round a boy who was good at playing the piano by ear. Although it was our usual practice to keep the pianos out of use in the sessions allocated for academic and quiet work, it was to everyone's advantage to allow Gordon to play over one or two tunes of his own composition on his arrival at school. Children are very understanding about this sort of thing. The group over which he presided operated in the afternoons, and as many instruments as possible were gathered together, orthodox and unorthodox, some of them worked by ingenious devices which the boys had rigged up. Sometimes the girls joined in as vocalists to the accompaniment thus provided. The tape-recorder figured prominently in this music-making, and the girls used it, too, for recording group and solo singing. Towards Christmas, carols were sung, played, and recorded. A number of girls and boys brought their sheet-music from home and kept up their music practice, and our music teacher gave one girl who had been a member of a church choir opportunities to practise the songs she had learnt. It made her feel that she had a future in which her accomplishment would again be used. Spontaneous singing, usually of pop songs, would break out, but sometimes hymns would be chosen and nearly everybody knew some verses by heart.

The gramophone and radio each played a dual part. Sometimes their use was reserved for classical music and concerts; sometimes a turn of the knob would bring on a popular song programme. Popular records, too, were taped and played back in season and out, if an alert ear were not kept open. We encouraged background music while the girls were sewing or the boys were modelling, for they listened to it in spite of themselves and heard fewer of the remarks which might otherwise have had an explosive effect. Popular music figures large in the adolescents' interest; a few profess to hate it intensely, protesting perhaps too much, but most of them love it inordinately. We had no desire to ban it, but could not agree to it being allowed to fill the whole day. During the last half-hour of each day, therefore, the youngsters were given the use of the gramophone for the records of their choice. They played them over and over again, sometimes just listening to them as they sat on the window bench, sometimes jiving and twisting to them.

For quite a number of children this last half-hour was what made afternoon attendance bearable, and its firm place in the time-table had an interesting history. In the early days of the school, the gramophone was a portable, hand-wound model, and the staff used records for the pleasure and interest they aroused in the psychotic and severely ill children who had an early morning period set apart for them. The other children heard the sound, and were attracted by it. At this time their musical activity consisted of attempts at group singing and a percussion band, really at a junior school level. The senior girls in this period were very difficult and unsettled, and it was hard even to keep them in the building. It was before we moved to our larger building, and they were cooped up in a tiny room behind a glass screen, yet such activity as we offered was their only alternative to being locked in the ward all day. We tried to introduce country dancing on the grass outside, but the sound of the music brought adult patients over, and certain young men made the out-of-door activity impracticable, particularly as the girls gave them every help. So we went indoors again but continued to use the gramophone. This brought a storm of protest from the male nurses who occupied the rest of the building, and it was finally proposed that we should use the gramophone only after 2.30 p.m. and only on two afternoons a week. We noticed, however, how the depression lifted on those two afternoons, and how much more willingly the girls settled down for the first part of the afternoon. By this time new and exciting records were appearing, and one of the boys begged to be allowed he hear his special favourites. Before long a new agreement was made by which we used the gramophone every afternoon for just half an hour, and the youngsters were told that they might bring their own records to put on. We bought certain records that were generally liked, using the balance of the staff tea fund for the purpose, plus any pennies paid by the children for a cup of tea during the afternoon. Later on, we were able to give this up, as many children owned so many records, and were very generous in lending them. The gramophone session continued after the move to the new premises. It was held in a special large room, and only those who wished to do so went in to listen.

To adult listeners some of the lyrics on the popular records seemed to be of little value, but the children used them to re-inforce meaning to themselves or to communicate meaning to others. One girl who was struggling to be accepted put on again and again 'I know what it's like to be lost in a storm.' 'I'll say I do,' she would add. Another girl rushed away from Max Bygraves's song 'Hands', and threw herself down to the ground in a storm of tears because she felt that she had had nothing in her life to thank God for. A boy would 'give' a tune to a girl – a device common of course, everywhere, but bringing peculiar comfort to these unhappy children. Other children found a technical satisfaction in listening intently to the backing or to the part contributed by a particular instrument, and they would catch one by the arm, and say: 'Listen.' Of course, the words of many songs were banal and the settings tuneless. Consequently, they turned the volume up too loud, so that they could hear nothing else and think of nothing else, and some of them seemed to clap, stamp, or dance as in a drugged reaction. It seemed as though they were thereby accepting the lulling and rocking of babyhood and, as they came through this re-experience, they found to hand the social pattern of dancing or sitting with a partner which helped them to keep growing desire within bounds.

At times jazz enthusiasts were included among our number; older youths who tended to scorn the crooners and whose music had the effect of separating them from the others. There was a demand for books on music, other than songbooks and tutors, e.g. on opera, jazz, ballet, and lives of classical composers, and they craved for magazines covering the meteoric life stories of young idols of the teenage world.

Closely linked with music was dancing, not only the jiving and twisting which was provoked by particular records, but ballroom dancing and a small amount of figure dancing. We were fortunate in having on the staff a gold medallist teacher of dancing, who offered her services freely to any boy or girl who wished to learn. She organized a group in which other members of the staff helped as well and she made opportunities for those who felt too shy or clumsy when in a group to learn with her by themselves. Her intuition and understanding were such that she could feel their bodily tensions and translate into words much of what they were fearing. Her expert knowledge and patience won their respect and confidence.

### Dramatic activities

Drama has already been referred to as part of the spontaneous play of some of the children, but it also had a definite position in our curriculum for at least three reasons: it stimulated creative activity, being so to say a livening-up agent, it provided a vehicle for the projection of feelings and ideas, and it was an excellent teaching medium in the hands of certain teachers.

Sometimes his spontaneous play enveloped the whole of the child's personality and was the only basis for a relationship between the child and the teacher. Boys would come in and curl up on a shelf in the cupboard, girls would ask for a blanket or one of the dressing-up fur coats and settle to sleep on the window bench. Tich made herself a cradle in the dressing-up wicker basket, to the confusion of the chaplain who chose that afternoon to visit us; Liz rolled under the table with a feeding bottle. This was their 'play' in which the teacher had to show concern by adding to the comfort, by giving a sweet at intervals, by noticing when the awakening was at hand, by verbalizing the child's desire to withdraw into babyhood and, at the right moment, by offering some incentives to growing up. The right moment often had to be found by trial and error, with the teacher quick to draw back again if he (or she) was arousing too much anxiety or, conversely, he had to be able to catch the flicker of an eye which might be the only indication that the child was ready to emerge from the chrysalis state. The incidence of sleep was interesting in a number of ways. Sometimes drowsiness was the result of medication and, if so, was reported to the doctor; sometimes it represented a wish to withdraw from an unwanted or over-demanding situation. But there were times, too, when hitherto over-active and highly suspicious children seemed to go to sleep to indicate that things had reached a stage where they could relax and place themselves, defenceless, into our hands.

In other children, play was active and voluble and had to be confined rather than extended. Norman and Rodney made up stories of cosh-and-run robberies and gathered an audience to watch them give realistic performances. They worked through a cycle of plots, developing a new theme only as they were ready to do so. They started with robbers outwitting the police, forcing an entry, binding and gagging householders, robbing banks, coshing, and leaving their victims to die. Then the police began to win; their method, too, being to cosh and leave their victims. The theme then changed to fires, with firemen effecting rescues, ambulances arriving to rush the injured to hospital, and doctors saving their lives. An attempt to get them to write down their plays met with only small success, but they would enthusiastically tape their dialogues, to which they added sound effects and in which they allowed pauses for the action to take place. Arlene organized court scenes and, in giving parts to other people, told them what to say, so that in effect she was in turn child, mother, policeman, magistrate, and probation officer. The words she put into their mouths were appropriate to each and showed her capacity for being objective about a situation which had been very painful for her.

Although other members of the group and the staff were sometimes drawn into this spontaneous play, the initiative usually came from one particular child. Members of the staff who carried out the actions ascribed to them were actors rather than co-authors of the plot. Thus they submitted to inspections and operations being performed on them by an efficient (child) doctor; became the ordered-about child of a domineering mother; or the stupid child of an angry teacher. When the same play had been repeated on several occasions the adult might feel it useful to introduce a twist into the pattern by standing up to the mother or becoming a successful pupil for a change, but would only do so if the child were ready for such a solution to the problem.

A number of children who needed help were those who, without withdrawing into the cupboard or sleep, had sunk into a pattern of safe-do-nothingness for whom the dressing-up basket and other props were insufficient stimulus, and whose apparent laziness made other children pass them over when looking for partners. One way of helping them was for the teacher to put on an act in front of a child for him alone, directing a flow of talk to him, asking advice, pleading for help to find a way out of a predicament. Another way was for the teacher to accept a part in someone else's play and to take the quiet child along, at least as a shadow, if not as a participant. These non-performers were catered for by the drama teacher in his organization of the official drama session where he used them as an audience. He used a modified form of charade; the audience were to try and recognize what was being performed or whose story was being portrayed. Thus, if *Hamlet* were to be the final subject, six small scenes, having no connection with *Hamlet*, or with each other, would provide the six letters. The seventh and final scene would be about *Hamlet*. Guessing right put the seal of success on their final watching.

This device was so skilfully prepared that hours of enjoyment were provided. Small groups of children would be primed for their part in the scenes, and information would be sought in books and encyclopaedias. Some children simply carried out what had been assigned to them, while others needed to be given only a hint and they would intelligently, even wittily, expand it into an apt situation; moving, tense, or hilarious.

Great ingenuity and care went into the preparations for these programmes. For a while we were able to set aside an afternoon each week during which the selected groups would work out what was to be presented but even so, it often happened that when the drama session itself was due, a leading actor would be too self-conscious to speak his part or would not arrive at all, either because stage fright or some hospital activity kept him away that day. To overcome these difficulties it became the practice to tape the dialogue and have it ready for an emergency. The dialogue was sometimes of the children's invention, but sometimes they read from plays, poems, or adapted narratives, and on the day itself the story was mimed to the taped dialogue. In this way scenes from history, from classical literature, from modern writers, from folk tales and traditions, were used. Old customs were re-enacted, such as maypole dancing, a pancake race, the Dunmow Flitch contest, beating the bounds, etc., and some children were found to have a wide fund of general knowledge on which they drew, and others became stimulated to read more about some of the subjects produced. Mention has already been made to the staging of a nativity play and to the making of rich clothes, etc. A lot of time was given up to making props for these weekly sessions: shields, crowns, swords, wigs, horses' heads, helmets, top-hats, and so on. Scenery was usually left to the imagination, helped by the arrangement of such furniture as we had. The items made were not put away for future use, as to go on playing with them gave great pleasure and prolonged the mood of the drama. The making of a costume would often spark off a good deal of play-acting quite apart from drama as a time-table subject. A hat particularly seemed to create a new personality, and it was quite an ordinary sight to see a boy wearing a hat while doing his lessons. Boys would dress as women with large busts and unborn babies, and girls paraded in long frocks and be-ribboned hats and fur coats as visitors; usually inspectors or committee members, who made critical or fulsome comments on everyone and everything. It became a great strain to have a programme ready for the drama session each week but, as the turnover of children was fairly quick, earlier programmes could be repeated with new mummers and changed emphasis. All the time things were happening which could be brought in to keep the programme alive and new, such as a child's sudden interest in puppetry, the arrival of a highly-skilled accordion player, a national or local

F

topic occurring like the budget or the Derby. It became the practice, too, to reserve one scene for emotional and/or abstract ideas, such as aggression, indolence, jealousy, etc. This often triggered off subsequent discussion or evoked confidences from the children and was also useful in supplying material for difficult letters. Sometimes, when it was not possible for the normal drama programme to be carried out, we would replace it by a game in which two groups operated in competition, one choosing and acting an adverb for the other to guess. The groups vied with one another to choose words which would be difficult to guess. More and more incidents and actions would be carried out to prompt the right answer, and the flow of ideas thus released was remarkable.

The whole school had the opportunity of attending the drama sessions which often proved to be times of great fun and strenuous activity as well as real teaching and learning periods, and children who at first sheltered in the audience were able more and more often to take part actively; first as one of a crowd, maybe, and later, as a main or solo character. Crowds had to be carefully handled and so did fights between two contestants. The actors often portrayed the characters too literally and lay about them much too heartily. One morning the shouts of a mob and the waving of cudgels was so realistic that a small band of nurses arrived from a nearby ward to rescue the school staff from a revolution. But more than one boy learnt control from pretending and, from stage aggression, learnt that aggression need not be unmanageable. The audience of these performances was far from passive. Everyone had to remain quiet, observe movement and dialogue, and search his memory to guess the answer.

The tape-recorder was a great boon. Play readings, B.B.C.-like interviews, music, street scenes, impersonations, and the remarks of unsuspecting visitors were all listened to with great interest. Two or three times the tape-recorder was used by a child who shut himself up with it in a closed room, as a confessional session in which he recounted his life story and revealed his fears and hopes to an imaginary audience, begging them to understand and to profit from the disclosure of incidents of which he had been ashamed or frightened. Several withdrawn children were stimu-lated into speech by being able to tape their own voices. Poor speakers had voice training practice via the tape. Tapes which were used only for drama items were kept separately and a big collection of scenes and subjects was built up.

A small puppet theatre and a number of puppets were available, as well as a set of 'Punch and Judy' puppets, complete with policeman, dog, and baby. Several children made a puppet of their own which they took with them when they left. Noel made a judge, and used him to pronounce sentence on others. We also made finger puppets representing a family, in which Mother on one hand could talk to the baby on the other, or right-hand 'Mum' could row with left-hand 'Dad'. The play and dialogue were usually spontaneous, but now and again the words would be stereotyped into a remembered pattern or even written down, and several sets of backcloth pictures were made.

Sometimes the puppet would be a human one, who would submit to being dressed up and led about, would speak as and when told to speak, and would walk, stand up, or sit as directed. The puppet's 'owner' usually showed great care and gentleness. Another substitute puppet was the dressmaker's dummy which normally lived in Mrs B's store cupboard. 'She' was often moved out into the room, a head provided by stuffing a hat and making a mask, and a variety of clothing was put on her. She also lived under a variety of names. Her most memorable was Florrie, given her by Lynne, who removed the body from its metal stand and placed it on the window bench. At first made to look full-busted, with a deeply plunging neck-line, drooping head with a cigarette hanging from the slack lips, Florrie went gradually through a series of transformations in which she became neater and more attractive. Her creator kept up a mocking commentary on Florrie's activities, but at weekends she was turned to look out of the window so that she should not feel lonely and afraid. At first no one dared touch her, but after some weeks it was noticed that Florrie's hair had dropped away, and finally she was returned, unwept, to the cupboard.

One other aspect of acting that might be mentioned was when one of the staff deliberately assumed a rôle in order to help a child. Verbal reflecting back and reflecting back in action were often used to lead on to further comment or self-criticism by the child. Rosa would say: 'Boo to you,' and put her tongue out. The teacher would simply reply, as nearly as possible in the same tone: 'Boo to you,' and put her tongue out. Rosa would stamp, and the teacher would stamp. Eventually Rosa would laugh saying: 'I am not like that,' knowing full well that her own behaviour, without any comment, had been mirrored back to her.

Sometimes a preview of an event would be staged to give a child confidence, as when a girl was scared at the thought of an interview with the Youth Employment Officer, or wanted to know the kind of thing she might expect if she took a certain job.

Altogether, drama served many purposes, and was indulged in on and off all the week, to say nothing of the uncontrived drama with its near catastrophic moments in which we all took part every day.

## Play and games

Organized outdoor games, running, and physical training came under the hospital's programme for out-of-school activities. In the school when outlets were needed for over-exuberant physical energy, lighter gamester balls were available, and large rubber balls were used outside. Games of tip-and-run were popular in the yard. Near the school we had a large tubular steel climbing-frame. It was designed for use by secondary school children but, after six months of the assaults made by our boys, so many faults began to appear that the makers replaced it with a specially reinforced model. The playing of seated table games was encouraged. Some boys and girls progressed to being able to become one of a group in this way, to play without cheating, or to endure being the loser. Games with playing cards were ultimately banned because gambling rings inevitably formed, but Chess, Draughts, Dominoes, various forms of Ludo, Snakes and Ladders, Monopoly, Scrabble, Lexicon, etc., all had their adherents, and paper games, chequers, and fiddlesticks kept individual children absorbed for long periods, as also did jigsaw puzzles. Some had favourite hobbies such as paper cutting and paper folding into manipulative models. Anything that engaged the attention, encouraged skilful co-ordination, and issued as either a tangible object or an intangible satisfaction (as from winning a game or making a picture), we found a place for in the child's programme.

## Fire and water

Our children all seemed to want to play with fire. For the majority it may not have held an attraction greater than for any children of their age. Since, however, a few had been fire-raisers on a scale which had been a danger to life and property, and since, in the hospital, fire was, with reason, the most dreaded danger, this interest caused the school staff a great deal of anxiety. We felt that its danger would be lessened if fire-making were allowed, but we felt that some reasonable precautions must be observed.

Some special day schools set aside an outside strip of playground in which the children may light fires in the later part of some afternoons. But what of those children who felt restless, destructive, or hyper-active in the mornings or on wet days? One of our difficulties was that we did not know enough about how the children were feeling when they wanted to light a fire.

The best we could do was to make our conditions. Indoor fires were to be kept small and only fed with rapidly consumed materials such as small pieces of paper and match-sticks; the fire must be made in the sink, in a non-inflammable container. If it was made on our formica-topped tables we objected when they were scorched but not to the fire itself. We praised those fire-makers who could keep the fire contained in the small space allotted to it and the children then began to take pleasure in controlling, as well as in making, a fire. Outside, there was an open shed in which we could permit fire-lighting on wet days and on fine days fires could be made in the yard or in the dustbin at the gate. At first, we stipulated that large pieces of wood were not to be used or wet material that made too much smoke. When one enterprising youngster noticed a heap of coal in the grounds and stoked the dustbin with this, we had to add hard fuel to the list of prohibited items.

A few of the children had nasty little sadistic habits, such as threatening to hold a lighted cigarette against a face. They would flick ash or cigarette ends or lighted matches into hair or clothing. We had to watch some of them very carefully but it was interesting to note that some of the most excited fire-makers became aware of the dangers and turned into the staunchest upholders of safety measures.

The hospital authorities arranged a huge bonfire with fireworks each year for Guy Fawkes night, and for days beforehand the boys would willingly pull a truck round the grounds to gather in rubbish of all kinds, broken-down furniture, dead branches, and garden waste. Mounting excitement made the days before the bonfire very difficult, and we forbade outright the letting off of fireworks within the school area, partly because of the danger, partly because the girls reacted so hysterically, and partly because we knew that, to obtain fireworks, some of the boys would climb the fence and steal from nearby shops. Eventually the boys were given a piece of wasteland known as 'The Dump', on which to play out of school hours, and there they were able to make large wood-fires without arousing anxiety in anyone.

There was a fire-alarm in the corridor of the school. The fire-hose was enclosed in a locked box. Occasionally the alarm glass would be broken: then the inter-communication telephones would ring, staff from the surrounding wards and the hospital fireman would arrive, and the greatest joy of all to the perpetrator would be the speedy arrival of one or more large red fire-engines with helmeted and booted crews.

Sometimes a class-room activity called for the use of fire as when Rodney built a model boat and bought an engine for it which needed solid fuel to provide the energy. Colin and others became interested in watching the power of steam force the lid off a tin part-filled with water, and rigged up a boiler over a small fire to demonstrate this. The rules about protecting the furniture and controlling the fuel were faithfully observed. We had two gas-stoves with ovens and boiling-rings, used mainly for cooking, but youngsters were allowed to use the heat in carrying out such experiments as melting down lead and burning out bamboo pipes. Sometimes they would choose to burn what they no longer wished to keep yet were determined that no-one else should have. This was the fate of John's farm model. Spread over a number of weeks, he had spent hours in its construction. He had no plan to copy, but his inventive mind thought of new features which he carried out quickly and competently. His interest in it arose at first from his wish to prove that he could bring an activity to a successful conclusion. At night he had it put carefully away, and invited his doctor over to see its progress. He bought a set of miniature farm animals and chickens, and painted the farm-buildings, fences, and trees. Then he would take it outside, burn part of it, say the barn, bring it in and renew it with an improved design. This was repeated with different sections several times, and his wish to remodel was given as his reason for burning it. After each renewal it was locked carefully away, until one day he removed the figures of the people and livestock, took the farm outside and watched it burn out completely. Balsa wood glue presented us with a problem at one period, for certain boys collected the near empty tubes and used them to burn out a lock on the ward, and we had to make a point of receiving back an empty tube before giving out a new one. In our whole history, however, there was no serious fire incident at the school itself.

Smoking presented a problem on its own. The official attitude to smoking varied from time to time, but, for the most part, smoking was forbidden on the wards and the possessor of cigarettes was punished. Many of the children had been quite heavy smokers before they came to hospital and everybody knew that, as opportunity offered, they would continue to smoke. They had no difficulty in getting cigarettes. Their parents and other visitors brought them in; when the children went on week-end leave, they brought cigarettes back; and adult patients were always willing to buy them for the children in the canteen. We decided that it was better to know what was going on than to drive it underground. So, although we did not approve of smoking, we did not forbid it, so long as it took place on the steps and not in the school itself. There were a few protests but most children found this rule reasonable. A smoker on the steps gave us a talking-point. We would discuss the cost of cigarettes, the injurious effect on health, the reasons why a child felt compelled to smoke, and what those who wished to might do to lose the habit. The staff did nothing to make smoking easier and they never smoked during the school day. They kept sweets or lumps of sugar on hand for the children who tried to cadge cigarettes or for those who were trying to give them up.

For some children water had even more fascination than fire and at times it had a surprisingly effective nuisance value. Many children used it in their regressive play. Polythene bottles with rubber teats were used for drinking and squirting. Sometimes a child (thirteen, fourteen or fifteen-year-old) would laugh and say: 'Let me be a baby. Hold the bottle and feed me.' Sometimes they would lie down comfortably with a bottle of warm tea and suck themselves to sleep. Or the water would be squirted out of a bottle held at hip level, a girl saying that she wished she were a boy, the boy laughing and calling attention to what she was doing. One boy, who didn't laugh, said that this was what his drunken father did. Mostly, they admitted that they were being babies. Occasionally the floor would be flooded, either when someone was 'cleaning' it, or when someone had deliberately let the sink overflow.

All the class-rooms in the school's second building had sinks with hot and cold water. This was a great help, since when there was no need to fetch water from an outside source there were fewer pretexts for leaving the room and a number of other troubles disappeared. Someone was always painting and he might use the table top itself as his canvas. He would flood it by pouring the water straight on to the powder paint. Whenever a boat was made, it had to be tested in the sink. The boys showed great ingenuity in constructing water-chutes and mechanical falling fountains, and even more in finding uses for lengths of rubber tubing. The girls often said that they longed for a hot bath, as they did not have much hot water on the wards. One aggressive and over-active girl became much more manageable when she was allowed to sit for a time with her feet in a bath of warm water.

Water was also used in cooking, but was most in demand when, as frequently happened, the girls had a washing-day. For a long time the ruling had been that, unless their families arranged for the laundering of their clothes, the children must wear hospital clothes and have them laundered by the hospital. These were redistributed each week quite indiscriminately, and pitiful their wearers looked in long, shapeless dresses and warm but ugly underclothes. The girls would, therefore, bring their own clothes over to school and wash and iron them. Favoured boys had their shirts washed for them, and others washed and ironed them for themselves and learnt to keep their trousers pressed with an iron and damp cloth.

Washing the walls also required the use of water; the walls were always in need of cleansing, from slogans mainly, sometimes from pictures whose originators had gone, and this washing was often a restitutive act in which one felt that the soul as well as the wall possibly emerged a little cleaner.

In the summer term the boys used the local swimming bath, and it was very interesting to note what a different aspect of himself might be presented by a boy through this other element – speed, freedom, confidence. Occasionally the girls were included in the swimming arrangements, but administrative difficulties always loomed larger in the female wards and girls could visit the baths only when a social worker or the psychologist was able to take one or two.

## BASIC SKILLS AND ATTAINMENTS

The amount of space already given to drama, music, art, etc., might suggest that we thought activities of this sort more important than the 'three R's'. But this was not so. For several reasons we gave time and attention to the basic skills. One was that to many people school means little more than reading, writing, and arithmetic. In fact, certain official visitors to the school expressed surprise at not seeing rows of desks with children sitting tidily at them, their heads bent over their books. And all that many of the children would say when asked about school was: 'I couldn't do sums', or 'My reading was all right'. Another reason was that for many of our children, this was their last chance for full-time schooling, as their discharge from hospital was going to come after they had passed the school-leaving age. Still another reason was that a fair number of children wanted it. Some had not found school work a difficulty and were anxious to make further advances or, at least, not to lose what they had acquired. Even some of the backward ones were able to admit regret at wasted opportunities and welcome remedial teaching. And, finally, it was encouraging to us to see a child lose his restless distractability and reach the stage where he could settle to work of someone else's choosing and persevere when it was difficult or even when it was dull.

When they first came, many could not settle at all to academic work. We were ready to wait and did not press them. Each child had his own 'tailor-made' programme. Some needed a much longer period of regression and 'pure' therapy than others. In time, the example of the more stable ones had its effect on the others. One interested child might fire the enthusiasm of a whole group. Even at their most regressed and resistant, the children would generally co-operate in doing tests of English and arithmetic. When they were a little more settled, work-books in which they could write the answer next to the printed question would hold their attention for a few minutes. After this, most children gradually achieved a longer span of attention and more effort could be demanded of them.

Although it was customary for the children, particularly for the girls, to say that they did not like arithmetic, after a time most of them were prepared to make at least a token effort in this subject. Some played with numbers at the infant school level, using the abacus and peg-boards. Others, who had genuinely missed out in mastering elementary processes, were glad to have step-by step tuition in the basic four rules and found great satisfaction in at last becoming competent. There were usually some who could accept further tuition in algebra and geometry and who were glad to keep up subjects which they hoped to take to examination level, and it was good for the staff to have mathematical problems to wrestle with. Plans drawn to scale or counted out on squared paper, measuring with a surveyor's tape, three-dimensional models made by following geometric constructions, and graphs, provided stimulation, as did exercises in technical drawing and books like *The Language of Shapes*. For those who needed remedial work or revision exercises the provision of a text-book was a tricky matter, for they were offended if the book proclaimed on its title page or in its foreword that it was for juniors. Some youngsters did not see why they should even bother to do any more sums; it was pretty clear that some of the older ones would not enter employment which demanded any skill with figures, and they would require only the ability to cope with everyday shopping, fares and postage and, accordingly, little was included in their programme. Others, however, who showed ability and who, moreover, would still be under statutory school-leaving age when they were discharged, were urged to keep up the knowledge they already had. They were asked to do revision exercises even if they felt incapable of making the effort to progress further. This 'ticking over' in the subject was important if they were to feel they had not lost ground on return to their own school. Others, refusing to show any interest in work done in a former school accepted an introduction to a topic new to them and worked keenly at, e.g. fractions, decimals, square roots, logarithms.

In addition to ordinary text-books we used a number of wide range test-papers in mathematics. Youngsters who seemed to us to be ready for it were gradually weaned from playing all the time by being asked to do a page of bookwork before they were provided with other materials which they wanted, and this demand was increased bit by bit. Although arithmetic was the least popular subject for many, there were some youngsters who wanted to concentrate all their time on doing mathematics. They achieved a good level of attainment in their work but were often obsessional in their preoccupation with numbers. Some children who had pronounced psychotic traits retained an ability to manipulate numbers; one boy excited admiration because he could correctly name without hesitation the day of the week appropriate to any given date. Another boy refused completely to occupy his mind with any calculation other than what he called mathematics of the fourth dimension.

Science as a laboratory subject was not possible, but a good deal of interest was, nevertheless, aroused by books like the Unesco report on science teaching in underdeveloped countries whose equipment had to be improvised. Several experiments were set up on similar lines and successfully carried out. Magnetism, electrical circuits, and radio were subjects which interested many boys and on which they were extremely knowledgeable. One boy was intensely interested in weather and well-informed about it, and most of them knew a good deal about aeroplanes and jet-propulsion. A film-strip on space exploration, rockets, etc., could be discussed with them in its technical jargon. Fortunately there was always one man on the staff who shared an interest in these things with the boys.

The weekly film-strip session enabled a large number of topics to be discussed in relation to various school subjects. Biographies of Columbus, Michelangelo, Grenfell, Captain Cook, Nelson, etc., the story of clocks and kitchens, and the Domesday Book, details for making books and puppets, copies of other children's pictures, books such as *Treasure Island, Oliver Twist, Aesop's Fables*, studies of bird and animal life, all stimulated reading and the search for further information. Some of the strips contained Bible stories, others were concerned with growing up and aspects of social life, from which a number of discussions arose, particularly among the girls.

There was usually sufficient interest in history, geography, and nature study for a number of attractive subject books to be made, greatly aided by illustrations from geographic magazines and B.B.C. pamphlets. Occasionally a boy would be found with a consuming interest in a period or aspect of history. Simon was attracted by the ruthlessly successful and studied Napoleon and Hitler in the greatest detail. Philip was more interested in political ideas and John studied costume. Simon was with us when the school was housed in the old school. His class-room door opened just across a narrow passage opposite the door of the office which was usually open. During his first few weeks Simon used to insist on the class-room door being left open too. He would place a chair up on a table, and with a greatcoat draped round his shoulders like a cloak, he would sit there, watching all that went on, from time to time uttering condemnations of what he saw and heard. An extract is given from Simon's play on Napoleon:

NAPOLEON: The uniform ... (*Bellamy picks up the coat. N gestures impatiently.*)

No. No. The breeches, man. (*Bellamy quickly hands N the breeches.*)

That's better. (*As he begins to put the breeches on, Ney, Murat, and Berthier come in, but seeing N is dressing, they begin to withdraw.*)

Come in, come in, my sirs. (*They enter and bow.*)

Everything must be hurried this morning. (*Busying himself about his coat, he turns to Murat.*)

Joachim, I expect you to have the cavalry ready to move off at eleven. (*Turning to Ney.*)

Your battalions will commence to march towards the Russians from Schevardino at nine. I require perfect discipline from all the troops. (*Turning to Berthier.*)

Sir, you and I will proceed to the forward lines as soon as I am ready – together we must set the pieces on the board. (*Berthier bows slightly.*)

BERTHIER: Your Majesty, I shall await your pleasure at Schevardino. (*He bows again and hurries out.*)

Latin was kept up by several youngsters who wanted to continue it for examination purposes, as were also French and German, but some children continued these simply out of interest in knowing a second language. A sporadic interest in Spanish was shown because several of the nurses came from Spain. English, however, provided the mainstay of the academic work. Language usage, grammar, comprehension exercises, spelling and vocabulary lists made up a good deal of the work, whereas spontaneous written work took the form of letters, stories and poems. Sometimes the story was deliberately intended to be autobiographical; sometimes incidents and feelings were projected under a thin disguise. Occasionally one of the children would contribute an item to the hospital magazine produced each week by the adult patients. Often the work was fragmentary but revealing:

B (1) I am an autumn leaf and I have been hanging from a twig for the last half-hour and have finally dropped. The tree I fell from is in a park and it was a chestnut tree, and I must say I'm glad I fell off because I was getting pushed around by those conkers. Now I can feel the wind blowing on my back and I'm sure my veins are sticking out. Ouch! That was the gardener brushing me aside with the other leaves but I don't want to go with them, I want to go on my own and explore.

(2) . . . The person who bought the pencil was a girl who was very imaginative, so when she saw how the pencil wrote, which was very unusual, she was delighted, but the pencil didn't like being pushed around, so he decided to run away . . .

s . . . Some trees not unlike willow trees overhang the pond and reflect in the water. There is another room joined on to the rest of the rooms. In this room you have to take your shoes off and walk barefooted as the floor. Unlike one of the other rooms, is made completely of glass, and the ceiling and the walls are also made completely of glass . . . This is a Utopia.

F All weapons of war would be abandoned and scientific progress would be for bettering the world rather than destroying it. The climate would be right in all parts of the world for the growing of abundant crops. There would be cures for diseases such as leukaemia where the sufferer has only a few years to live. All families would be united and orphans found homes.

J A distant clock chimes twelve times – midnight. In the town the lights still flicker, a few voices are still to be heard; but on the outskirts, in the churchyard, all is hushed, all is still. The tombstones, blanched and pale, stare vacantly up at the night sky, some slimy with moss and speckled with a few withered anemones. The grass, overgrown and uncared for, bends softly to the wind as though in prayer. A statue of Our Lady, pitifully drained of colour and with one arm broken off, stands surveying this human burial ground as she is doomed to do until she crumbles into nothingness.

G . . .

WITCH: Take this. (*She gives Dr Hawk a small cardboard box.*)

DOCTOR: What is it?

WITCH: Powder. Wasps' stings. (*She picks up a small bottle and gives it to Dr Hawk.*)

Take this bottle of child's blood and mix it with the powder. (*As she is giving it to him it falls to the floor and the contents are spilled.*)

O may all the cows born tonight be cross-eyed! Why didn't you take it? Every drop is spilled.

DOCTOR: I can't see it in this dim light.

WITCH: I'll get some more and you shall pay me for it.

DOCTOR: Where will you get it from?

WITCH: You are visiting Mr Kio, I believe, who is suffering from overwork.

DOCTOR: Yes, but how did you know?

WITCH: The moon told me. Give Mr Kio this pill of frog's brains and send him to bed. (*She gives him a pill from a bottle.*) He has a little dark-haired girl. See that the girl is left alone by herself. I will do the rest.

Sometimes attempts were made at writing verse as an exercise, but now and again poems were the spontaneous outpourings of thoughts and feelings, usually successfully conveying a mood or emotion.

Reading matter ranged from comics to the *Spectator*, from 'Look and Say' reading cards to reference books packed with technical information. An intelligent child who had for years resisted being taught to read might suddenly see the need for it. It might be a letter from a girl friend that decided him – after months in which he had had his parents' letters read to him.

Every child identified himself very strongly with his own group. The groups were family size and their central figure – the teacher – was a parent-substitute. For the child too timid to venture beyond it the group was a place of safety and it was also a setting in which he ran no risk in acting out his anger, resentment, or jealousy. When he reached the stage of daring to leave his sanctuary, he still needed it to come back to. In time, as he became more secure and more able to trust the father- or mother-figure, he would learn to tolerate and, sometimes, even to welcome into his group a child who belonged elsewhere.

Eventually a day might come when he would join with two or three other children to work out some project and carry it through. As stability, confidence, and perseverance increased and as violent outbursts became less frequent, he would begin to apply himself seriously to academic work. Then, soon afterwards, it would seem to us that he was not going to need the shelter of our environment much longer and that the time was coming for his discharge.

Properly speaking, it was not for us to say whether or not a child was ready to leave, but the doctors usually consulted us and paid great attention to our observations and records. On those occasions when we thought the right thing was to keep the child in the school, although he was being discharged from medical care, they were ready to help us by making the necessary official recommendations. They consulted us, too, about the sort of work the children ought to try to get. We were all agreed on the importance of building up the child's confidence and self-esteem. When we suggested a job where the child would fit in and be happy, even if it was far below his capabilities, they would agree. They would leave to us, however, the task of soothing the ruffled feelings of the parents and talking them out of their disappointment. Somehow, we were quite successful at this and got a good deal of satisfaction from finding that our last task as parent-substitutes was to help re-establish a good relationship between the child and his real parents.

# 5
# The teachers

So far only passing reference has been made to the teachers, but this does not mean that I did not value them or recognize the contribution each made in his or her own way. Only people of exceptional stamina could have stood up to the work, and only those who were outstandingly selfless and outstandingly patient could have been sustained by results so meagre and so slow in coming.

The job of the school staff was never very clearly stated. We occupied the children with interesting and useful activities but we were not occupational therapists. We kept watch over them during the hours in which they were committed to us but we were not child-minders. We were experienced with young people and we were students of their development but we were not psychotherapists. In the complex set-up of our Unit the resolving of the children's difficulties depended on all its members, not on one section alone, though we felt that as teachers we had an important part to play. We belonged as much outside the hospital as in it. We dealt with matters that had occupied the children before they came to hospital and that would occupy many of them after they left us. We were able to leave the children alone and yet maintain a protective supervision over them. We made it possible for them to verbalize their feelings in a way that was of immediate value to us in our dealings with them and was probably going to be of worth to them in the future.

Probably the teacher who had the hardest time in the school was the 'extra' teacher who replaced each of the others as they took their term-time leave. No matter how difficult the children had made life for their own teacher and no matter how much they liked the substitute as a person, as soon as she came to take over their group, they projected on to her all the resentment they felt at being deserted by their own teacher. Some children could not tolerate staying in the room when their teacher was away; some would take refuge in the office or in a room where they had a friend; some would refuse to come to school until he or she returned.

A skilful substitute might overcome their hostile feelings and get herself accepted, but her very success changed the character of the group. Activities that had flourished with their own teacher were laid aside even when he had made every preparation for them to be carried on. New interests were taken up, only to be dropped as soon as he returned. On his return the children would make a show of lavishing affection on the substitute teacher, while being quite off-hand with him and saying, e.g. 'Oh, you're back are you? Why didn't you stay away?' or 'We don't want you, it's better with her.' The original teacher would have to go through all that the substitute had endured, while she, poor thing, was going through it all over again with the next group.

If, however, the substitute teacher could stick it out, things improved. A group that saw her for the second or the third time was less suspicious and unco-operative and might even dimly appreciate the fact that she was making it possible for them to continue as a group throughout the term. Her colleagues certainly valued her. She was the only teacher who knew every group, and so saw things slightly differently from the rest of us.

The permanent group teacher guided the activities of the class-room, creating in it a milieu in which the children could learn. He had to gauge the mood of each child and support the waverer or offer sympathy to the defeated. The teacher would test the progress of a child by slightly delaying his response to a demand and he would encourage those pursuits which seemed to be contributing to a child's intellectual or social improvement. He also presided over the resources of the class-room and did his best to see that each child had the materials or equipment he needed. Sometimes, however, an utterly unreasonable request would be made. The teacher would then discuss it with the child and try to understand what lay behind it. If the child was simply 'trying it on', the other teachers would be informed so that the child could not play one of us off against the other.

The group teacher had the oversight of each child's programme and decided how much pressure could be brought to bear on the child and for how many hours per day or week to expect him to attend. In particular, it was the teacher's job to build up the child's confidence and bring him to the stage where he would stick at a piece of work, even if he found it difficult.

The teacher had to be continually ready to reappraise his plans and change his approach. In dealing with our children flexibility was only less important than equanimity. Flexibility was equally important in team-work with the other teachers. Since each teacher was a specialist at something, if a child wanted help with a particular subject, he would want to go from his own group to another. Thus one or two who belonged to Group A might go to Group B for woodwork, and one from Group B to C for Latin and so on. This meant that each group might change its composition several times in the course of the day and no teacher had one unchanging set of children sitting tidily behind closed doors. Some teachers found this untidy structure too much for them. But this freedom to go away at times from the group to which they belonged gave the children a sense of security. 'They shall go out and find pasture' but only when there is a safe base to come back to.

The children needed and respected people who 'knew' and who knew how to communicate their knowledge, whether of music, drama, technical drawing, or mathematics. They were always anxious for reassurance that their teachers really 'knew' – i.e. that they had qualifications that were recognized outside the despised hospital school. They would ply the staff with questions about the examinations they had passed and about their work and position in other schools. They needed to believe that their teachers were worthwhile in order to feel worthwhile themselves.

In short, the teacher had to fulfil two functions, one passive, the other active, each the complement of the other. He had to see all and hear all – no easy task when the place was full of action and noise – he had to keep his channels of communication open all the time and, when giving his attention to one child, not let himself be bogged down into the interests of the moment to the exclusion of the needs of other children. No more than a smile, a word, a raised eyebrow might be necessary to indicate his interest, but each child had to know that he was observed and held in mind. In the same way, the teacher's ears had to be open so that, later, reference back could be made to something a child had said. The discussion was often days, or even weeks, later, but this lapse of time did not seem to matter so long as the child knew that what he had said had been noted.

In the second place, the teachers had to be available when needed, giving protection to those who sometimes needed it, showing firmness to others. The protection was not only good for the oppressed but also for the fears of the oppressor. Listen to Kahlil Gibran, when the judges of the city ask the Prophet to speak to them of crime and punishment:

'And this also, though the word lie heavy upon your hearts;
The murdered is not unaccountable for his own murder,
And the robbed is not blameless in being robbed.
The righteous is not innocent of the deeds of the wicked,
And the white-handed is not clean in the doings of the felon.
Yea, the guilty is oftentimes the victim of the injured.
And still more often the condemned is the burden bearer for the guiltless and unblamed.
You cannot separate the just from the unjust and the good from the wicked;
For they stand together before the face of the sun even as the black thread and the white are woven together.
And when the black thread breaks, the weaver shall look into the whole cloth, and he shall examine the loom also.'

Difficult words to understand, but there were times when we could see exactly what they meant: when quiet non-participation was more aggressive than assault would have been. On many of these occasions we found it easier to come to terms with the conscious exploitation of the weak by the strong than with the apparent apathy of the weak who, nevertheless, placed themselves with uncanny accuracy in the way of the strong.

We had to be on the lookout for bullying all the time. The psychotic children were easy game. Children who showed that they were frightened also invited attack and there is a passive type of child who seems to be a born victim. The staff could never turn a blind eye to what was going on. Although, as far as possible, they acted to deflect aggressors and to provide them with alternative outlets, they were ready to intervene to prevent bullying and the children knew this. The usually gentle and affectionate behaviour of the teachers to the children had, in the long run, a good influence on the children's behaviour to one another, but the sovereign remedy for bullying, as for all other problems, was to bring it into the open in group discussion. Teachers, of course, participated and if a child was too withdrawn or too intimidated to speak for himself, a teacher would speak for him. Children used to criticize teachers in these discussions and reacted violently against what they regarded as 'unfair'. They showed bitter resentment if it seemed to them that an adult was 'taking sides', but were quite ready to allow a teacher to act as the mouthpiece of the tongue-tied.

In addition to the tasks undertaken by all the teaching staff, the Head had special responsibilities. She was the representative of the school in its relationships with people outside it – not only with all the departments and the different professions within the hospital, but also with the County Education Department, the Ministry of Education, and various official committees (see Chap. 6, p. 96). Just as she represented the school to these people beyond it, so she represented these outsiders to the school. She had a responsibility to the staff as well as to the children. Also she was the school's administrator to the extent of seeing that equipment and stock were supplied, that the fabric of the building was maintained, that it was as little damaged as possible, and that damage was made good.

While the academic aims of the school and the goals of social behaviour were those agreed by the whole staff, it fell to the Head particularly to see that they were always kept in mind.

To the staff she was primarily a colleague but she had the ultimate responsibility. It was she who, when necessary, spoke the final word to the children.

Another of the Head's tasks was to be co-ordinator, and she had a special task when resignations occurred, minimizing the shock of loss, and, when a new colleague arrived, easing the adjustments that were called for. The adjustments were, of course, on both sides and time had to be given to let newcomers feel their way into the new situation and reveal their special strengths. They needed support and encouragement when, after the first flush of novelty had worn off and the uglier aspects of the work were seen, feelings of inadequacy and depression threatened to become dominant. They would also need scope for their talents and acceptance of their idiosyncrasies. Hierarchical attitudes are prone to persist between head teacher and staff, but it seemed odd that this should be so where acceptance was the keynote of the attitude to the children. The last thing I wanted was that acceptance should appear to be a technique for dealing with sickness rather than the basis of respect for individuals.

In relation to the children the Head had a varied rôle. Often it must have seemed that she was just there, in the office with the door open, in the corridor, or moving from one room to another. But the children felt that she was always accessible, always interested. At times she was the recipient of overflowing love, at other times she was the object on which they vented their hate.

Our practice was to keep the staff-room as the one place to which the children were never admitted and we met there at the mid-morning and lunch-time breaks. We talked mainly of the children, of our own home affairs, of the books we had read, or theories to which we were inclined. In the main, we were able to talk to each other freely, commenting and questioning and enjoying the mutual support which this give and take provided. In addition, we had a formal staff meeting once a week at which conference news and general topics of policy were discussed. We discussed two or three children each time so that each one would have been considered in the course of the term, but giving priority to those who were likely to be discharged or to those who were presenting us with some specially difficult problem.

There were times when we felt cut off from the rest of the educational world, overlooked in the hospital, and discouraged in our own group. Then it was that a visit from our own understanding consultant or the right sort of visitor was a godsend.

It was also a help to discuss fully what we were doing and what we were aiming at. Work of this intensity depleted us of vital energy and there were times when the weight of the aggression, sorrow, and despair made it almost impossible to cope with even the physical demands of the situation. But there was the other side of the picture, too; times when we could see gaiety and goodness in the children, and wonderful days when we felt we had achieved something.

The children were aware of the attitudes of the adults as children are in a family. We always tried to let them see that we were for them and not against them. When, for instance, a child was trying to play one adult off against another, he and the two teachers would get together and comb the matter out, not so that a two to one verdict should result but so that all three should reach an agreed conclusion and be clear about the way in which it had been reached. The children felt supported by the staff, but saw how the staff supported one another. They saw that adults, although they might differ in outlook just as much as children did, could usually settle their differences peacefully and amicably.

During the years under review the school was the only part of the Unit in which men and women worked together. Only once, and then for a short period, was there a woman doctor. The male doctors may have provided the girls with father-figures, but there was a sad lack of mother-substitutes for the boys, in whose wards the nurses were also male. Apart from the school, the only women the boys met were the psychologist, the social worker, the lay psychotherapist, and a woman helper in the ward to look after the boys' clothes, but fortunately a warm person in whom they liked to confide.

We felt it was a good thing that there were always teachers of both sexes and that there always were open dealing, good-humour, and mutual respect in our relationships.

# 6
# Relationships with the outside world

From the school's point of view everyone other than teachers and pupils was an outsider but this was not the point of view of various groups of people who were either interested in the work of the school or who were concerned with its management. The doctors, nurses, and others who belonged to the Unit had a special responsibility for the children and we had to remember that the school's control over them was no more than partial. For instance, all routines associated with bedtimes, meals, clothes, medication, etc., were arranged by the wards and the ward staffs were part of a fairly rigid hierarchy.

The boys' ward was controlled by a charge nurse, with junior nurses to carry out his orders. At first relations between this ward and the school were stiff but, later, when the régime on the wards became more relaxed, a charge nurse was appointed with whom the school staff could work easily. The girls' ward was in the charge of two sisters who, too, at the beginning ran it with rigid and rather inhuman discipline. For a long time the girls were locked in, only a few ever being allowed to leave the ward unescorted. Later this, too, became an open ward with a much warmer atmosphere. In both wards a number of the assistant staff were from overseas and spoke very little English. This was not, however, a complete disadvantage to the children for they could take these nurses under their protection and feel slightly superior to them.

It will no doubt be clear that the school did not always present a calm, well-ordered picture to visitors. Although things changed eventually with a new generation of nurses, in the days when the ward discipline was strict and inflexible, we tried to run the school without nurses in attendance. Some nurses who escorted children to and from the school often felt impelled to intervene, checking and criticizing children who were behaving in a way that we were allowing. The children talked about the school in the wards and relayed to us such statements as 'You can do what you like in the school,' and 'The school's a circus, anyway, that's what the nurses say.'

People such as the psychologist, the lay psychotherapist, and the psychiatric social worker, allies though they were, sometimes in the early days seemed to be working against us as, e.g., when they sent for a child just at the moment when we most wished for his presence in the school. Later, we seemed to reach a better understanding with them. Perhaps it was that we adjusted ourselves better to the reality of being a hospital school.

We enjoyed excellent relations with the three consultants who during the school's existence had charge of the Adolescent Unit. Junior doctors were not, on the whole, quite so easy to work with, though there were many who became firm friends and helped overcome the disapproval the nurses felt for our methods.

Nurses and doctors from other parts of the hospital had no direct concern with the school but, since they regarded it as either a show place or as a chamber of horrors, most of them made some pretext for visiting us and bringing their friends. We had many visits from psychiatrists, psychologists, social workers and teachers, often from overseas, and also from nurses in training in our own and other hospitals.

Apart from these, there were more formal relationships with the various authorities who had some responsibility for the running of the school. In common with all schools in the state educational system, we came under the local (County) education authority, who staffed, equipped, and financed the school, and the Ministry of Education (now Department of Education and Science). In addition, as a hospital school, our premises, heat, light, water, etc., were provided by the Hospital Management Committee, who were inclined to believe that the school was theirs. In fact, very soon after the school was set up, a Governing Body was formed with members drawn from the County Education Committee and from the Hospital Management Committee in equal numbers.

All these bodies were entitled to pay official visits, the Ministry of Education always giving us notice of their coming, the others

descending on us without warning. Sometimes a whole committee would come, sometimes (fortunately) they would send two
representatives. The children saw little difference between official
and unofficial visitors and, while the visitors were with us, would
make a special effort to display comparatively orderly and near-
orthodox class-room behaviour. But, as soon as the visit was
over, they would explode with resentment and accuse the staff of
'bringing people to look at them like animals in a zoo'.

To the staff the official visits were the greatest strain. These
visitors were, of course, entitled to criticize. Many of them, in
spite of our explanations, had little understanding of the children's
needs or of our aims. Some failed to grasp that an experiment was
going on and expected to see children sitting in orderly rows who
rose and said a deferential 'Good Morning'. One member asked
how a hole had been made in the office door. When the teacher
said that a broken door was at least better than a broken leg, she
was asked not to be facetious. On another day a Committee
arrived soon after a big effort of restitution had been made. The
teachers were complimented on the improved condition of the
walls; obviously discipline was better. When the teachers explained what had happened, they were rebuked for allowing time
meant for academic instruction to be used for cleaning walls.

The meetings of the Governing Body were the worst strain for
the Head. She had always to be present and give a report. This
often met with a good deal of hostile criticism. The physician-
superintendent of the hospital, who was a member, gave little
support, while the consultant in charge of the Unit who was in
sympathy with the school and could be quite persuasive, was only
occasionally invited to be 'in attendance'. However, in time the
attacks became less virulent. Some members of the Committees
acknowledged that, even if we were misguided, at least we were
sincere. Others came to see that, however appalling children's
behaviour might be, they were desperately in need of help and
affection. A few members even paid unofficial visits and took
trouble to get to know individual children.

Most of the children, however, had few outside contacts and
they set great store by their rare visits home and by visits to the
hospital from their parents. The majority of parents, when they
came, were eager to meet someone in authority to ask about their
child's progress. They wanted to speak about the anxieties and
disappointments that the child's illness had aroused and they

wanted to unburden themselves of the many stresses and strains in their own lives.

When a child was admitted, the psychiatric social worker interviewed the parents to obtain as full a history as possible of the case. The psychiatric social worker then kept in touch with the home. When the time came for the child's discharge, she prepared the family for his return or made plans for him to live elsewhere. As a rule the doctor also interviewed the parents, at least at the beginning and end of the child's stay. The school staff took no part in these exchanges and had a chance to meet the parents only if a child asked if they might come and see the school. We were very glad of any opportunity to get to know the parents but we could not allow them to penetrate further into the school than the office. It was not only that we were afraid that our seemingly disorganized class-rooms would affect parents in the same way as they did most other visitors, but we felt that it would be particularly distressing to them to see their own child in this setting. We also wanted to spare other children distress. To see one child with his parents brought to the surface all their feelings of deprivation and rejection.

Once we had met the parents they often made overtures towards a closer relationship with the teachers. They would write or telephone for an appointment or ask for a specific teacher to give them some piece of advice. We would never agree to seeing them without the approval of the doctor and the social worker, but some parents seemed to prefer to confide in the teacher.

The children, much as they looked forward to seeing their parents, were often unhappy afterwards. They built up such hopes in fantasy and tended to expect the impossible. The reality often left them disappointed and depressed, and then they would project on to the staff their feelings of resentment and bitterness. The staff, often enough, felt equally depressed and disappointed by visitors. They suffered for the children and from the children's reactions. With few exceptions, visitors were hostile critics. However much we might tell ourselves that we knew better than they, it was hard not to lose confidence in our own beliefs.

These moods were, fortunately, short-lived. We could generally regain our equanimity, our sense of humour, and our sense of purpose by a full discussion at a staff meeting. And our closest colleagues helped and supported us. Each of the three consultants who in turn had charge of the Adolescent Unit believed in the way we ran the school and would come to our aid when we were in danger of losing our belief in ourselves. They were always ready to defend us and to interpret us to scoffers. The clinical psychologist interpreted what lay behind many of the children's actions and so helped us to understand and accept our unhappy pupils and, sometimes, to see some value in our work.

Each of the three consultants had been experienced in child psychiatry. The second was also a paediatrician and a member of a family famous in the world of progressive education. Before he left the Unit he prepared a blue-print for the future of the Unit, laying down its needs in accommodation, numbers, ratio of staff to children, medical staffing, and so on. His successor worked to get this put into effect and conditions were approaching the ideal when, with very little warning, the whole thing was brought to an end.

In the earlier years we found ourselves much concerned about what was likely to happen to children who had been discharged. If the boys and girls discharged were over statutory school-leaving age it presumably became the duty of someone in the area of the children's home to help them find employment. Those under fifteen had to return to school. We were more and more convinced that these were questions which should be asked, and at least tentatively answered, before discharge. For some children there might be little problem, but for others, such as those who had failed in a particular school, those who had no real hope of support from their family and needed hostel facilities, or those who would profit from a specific training course, there was much exploratory work to be done. The social worker had usually co-ordinated the questions asked by conference members, and had maintained close contact with us in the school where aptitudes and abilities, or lack of abilities, had been revealed, and a very valuable aspect of the conference work as time progressed was the carefulness with which placing after discharge was considered. Unfortunately, two big areas remained to be dealt with, the pro-vision of an after-care clinic attached to the Unit, and some kind of follow-up of the boys and girls who had been discharged. Follow-up work was done systematically in the first five years, when the psychiatrist who founded the Unit was in charge and doing research into juvenile schizophrenia, but since then we had been obliged to rely only on such information as we received from letters, telephone calls, and visits made to us by the boys and girls themselves. Occasionally we received chance information from workers in other places.

Often we have been asked how successful our work has been. We know that some of our boys and girls have had to go directly from us to other institutions, perhaps for life-long supervision and care, or that others have been sent there later. We know that others have returned home and, with the help of their families, schools, and other agencies, have made a new start. Some of these, we feel, will continue to do well, but others may require specialist treatment every now and again as crises recur, but on the whole they will be equal to the normal demands of community life. It is better, perhaps, to think in terms of progress rather than of cure, and if the criterion is that they are able to live outside the special environment provided by an institution, the quality of the community in which they try to live will also be a factor in their success. It might also be said that their time with us, while not in itself effecting a 'cure', made them readier and more able to accept help from some other agency further along the line.

# 7
# The children

Our Unit was originally intended, as has already been said, for psychotic children but, in fact, we had a great variety of difficult children of whom only a few were psychotics. But they had an effect out of all proportion to their number. The other children jeered at them and called them 'dossie' or 'dopey' and seemed to despise them. It seemed to us, however, that this show of contempt concealed a very great fear and we thought that the presence of these utterly disintegrated personalities made the others uncomfortably aware that they, too, were nearly as much at the mercy of inner disruptive forces. We could only hope that, by showing concern for the psychotics, we could indirectly comfort their tormentors. The psychotic children needed love that was demonstrated by caresses and physical closeness. By giving this sort of tenderness to the disintegrated we felt we were helping in some small way to dispel the fear of disintegration in the others.

In the days when we were occupying the old school we set aside an hour for the most disintegrated children in which they could do what they wanted to do, either alone or with the teacher of their choice. Activities such as baking, painting, listening to records, using percussion instruments, and dressing up were provided for them. They enjoyed water, sand, clay, and feeding bottles and were delighted to be able to move from room to room. They were able to exhibit their symptoms, even rocking, masturbation, and biting at their clothes, without criticism. We tried to encourage them in any skill in which they showed an interest and we tried to increase their awareness of others. Occasionally we were rewarded, when one of them made a friendly overture to another child.

Perhaps a manifestation of the split in their personalities was the way in which they referred to themselves. Many never used the first person singular but spoke of themselves as 'She' or 'You' or 'The Boy'. When Marie wanted to have something, she would say: 'She dreamed she could have . . ., she did.' Others seemed to think of themselves as two people. Frances, e.g., insisted that she had a twin, Dora, and that Dora did all the bad things. She painted a picture of Dora which she put on the wall and when she looked up at Dora, we knew that there were troubles ahead. Rosa, in her moods of disturbance would use her three-part name or, when she knocked things over or made a great mess, would say: 'It wasn't me, it was Rosa C . . . J . . ., the bad one.' Rosa was typical of those children with a long history of defective behaviour who were admitted for diagnosis. At the beginning she was aggressive and noisy, occupying herself by cutting or tearing newspaper or by interfering with the others and damaging their possessions. One day she gave one of the others a vicious slap, and immediately said: 'It wasn't me. I didn't hit Hilda, did I?' When her teacher said that perhaps Rosa couldn't bear to know that she had hurt Hilda, Rosa said: 'I hate Hilda because she is a ballet dancer.' She went on to talk of ballet frocks with lots of frills and was asked if her mother had made her one. She shouted fiercely: 'No, you must have a young lady's dress, not that silly nonsense,' and then, equally excitedly: 'I will not put up with it . . . The beating you will get.' Asked who was always so angry, she replied: 'Do you mean Miss L?' (the name was not known to us). 'What had Miss L done to her?' 'Not to me, to Rosa C . . . J . . .' Miss L, it appeared, had hit her, but when she ran away to tell her mother (here she became very anxious and indistinct), her mother had 'sloshed her in the face'. Later that morning the teacher (at Sebastian's) to whom she told this story, in a game with another child, pretended to cry and said: 'Don't hit me, Miss L.' Rosa came at once and asked what was the matter. The teacher used a phrase that Rosa herself often used when in distress: 'Who will comfort me?' 'I will,' said Rosa, 'Come and sit in a nice chair. You are upset aren't you? Were you crying for me?' The teacher said 'Yes', and when Rosa asked 'Why?', said: 'Well, because I like you.' 'Yes, you do don't you?' said Rosa. From this moment we felt we were on terms of understanding with Rosa. She still had her moods and her moments of disturbance, but we could tease her and pull her leg. After a time she reached a stage where she could accurately write all the figures from nought to nine and where she would set herself sums. In these a number was to be added to itself, e.g. ten plus ten, two plus two, etc., and she could do them correctly. She made a beginning with a simple reading book and her behaviour became better. Just at this moment, she was moved to a subnormality hospital.

Another group who were regarded as defective were those who were so withdrawn that they were largely mute, almost it seemed at times, because they could not bear to discharge openly their intense hostility. They were, however, aware of all that went on around them. Judy was like this. Apparently she had begun to display this behaviour early, and had not been weaned from it during her primary school days. She had learnt almost no skills and she was termed severely subnormal. In the class-room she would sit alone at a table pushed against a wall, her back to the rest of the room, her arms on the desk to shield what she was doing from view, and her hair falling to hide her face. She had learned to make a written copy of a printed page and had a well-formed, controlled hand. Difficult many-pieced jigsaws she completed with speed and accuracy. When she was finally tempted away from the side table to join a painting group she began by always producing the same sort of picture, of a round face surmounted by a conical cap above a round body, armless and legless, like a tumbling toy that rights itself. She was aware of everything that went on in the group and her eyes gleamed when insulting jeering language was used to the staff or aggressive acts took place in the room. But whatever was going on she would remain firmly seated on her chair, scarcely uttering a sound.

Her delight broke through into loud laughter one day when in the early morning session the two men teachers turned up a table and put on an act of two naughty babies quarrelling in a perambulator. She began to move about more freely and became much attached to one of the men, allowing him to tease her a little. But she used to give sly pinches to other children and became smoulderingly angry when told she must not do so. She was not limited to the early session but came to school all day, although no pressure towards academic work was put on her. It was felt she needed to play, to experience something of the gaiety of a good infancy, in music, rhymes, and stories, to indulge her whims, and to find a way out of her fortress. Judy occupied herself in all sorts of ways; learned to use the sewing machine and to make herself skirts; to cook; to make felt stuffed animals; to make baskets and many other things extremely well. Gradually the occupations became a little more aligned to orthodox school-work – she made scrap-books on particular topics, copied recipes into a note-book and learned to recognize them, and she would watch word games. She now responded frequently with smiles and laughter. However, she would not yet ask for help but sat and waited for it to be noticed that she needed scissors, or a pencil. She identified with the teacher, however, in calling out to other girls who were on the point of making mistakes in their work, or told the teacher that someone had taken the sugar or played some other trick. The one period in which she permitted herself any physical activity was during the last half-hour of the school day when the gramophone room was open. Judy would untie the belt of her teacher's white coat and run down the corridor with it, inviting pursuit. When the belt had been recovered she would take it again and again and, at times, would put the belt into her bag and go off with it.

At about the time that Rosa left the Unit the doctor suggested that Judy was a mental defective and that she, too, should be discharged. Since Judy continued to refuse all psychological testing, there was no psychologist's report to support either the doctor's view that she was subnormal or that of the school staff that she had a fair measure of intelligence which was becoming more and more accessible. Since she was still only thirteen, we were very anxious that she should continue in the school, to which she had now become accustomed. Fortunately, her home was only about an hour's journey away. The Education Authority agreed to pay her fares, and it was arranged that Judy should live at home but attend the school daily.

At this point we transferred her to the older girls' group and told her that she was expected to begin to read and to reckon like the others. She accepted this move, and over the next eighteen months covered a most rewarding programme of work; learning to read stories, to fill in elementary English work-books, to master the four rules in arithmetic and to apply them to money, and to cut out and use a paper pattern. Working consistently to the full capacity of an eighty to ninety I.Q. level, she was tidy and clean in her person. She continued to do jigsaw puzzles, to make felt toys and to play with the teacher's belt. However, she continued to be rather sparing of conversation, but she showed her emotions more freely, and made friends with a very outgoing girl. Suddenly, for some days, she played truant, travelling to and from home on the same buses as usual, but going on past the hospital and presumably into the neighbouring town for the day. When she returned to school again, she would give no explanation of what she had been doing or why, and it remains a mystery whether her lapses represented anxiety or initiative. She began to look forward to growing up and, when she reached her fifteenth birthday, decided to leave school and go to work. Her first job lasted only a week, but at her second attempt, at a factory paying piece-rates, she settled down well and earned a living wage.

Others coming to the Unit had reached adolescence before developing a psychotic illness, and some of these often retained their skills in reading, writing, and number, but their fantasies predominated, and we wondered how best to deal with these fantasies. At times it seemed right to enter into them; pointless as well as cruel to explode them. When, e.g. Marina, a girl who had had a pre-frontal leucotomy, said fearfully that a bear was pressing against her leg, her teacher opened the door and told the bear to go outside. She then talked with Marina about things that frighten us and, as Marina recalled how she had loved her Teddy-bear, she became relaxed and happy for a brief interlude.

Some children with marked psychotic features retained enough drive and energy and a sufficient outer semblance of normality to be accepted by the other children. The energy, however, was not directed to an end and their communications were bizarre. Examples are given from the writings of J (a boy) and P (a girl):

J   To give you a general outline of how different kinds of weather have affected me, here is a chart and incidents. *Hot*. It could make me go lazy and send me somewhere else than where I was. My life at times was full of screens, sometimes when I knew the weather was ripened for two persons to continue the ripening for me, I was catapulted to where moors and all ingredients were perceived. I was a third person. If the weather had been opposite and I had corresponded to it, then by hypnotical powers it might change late in the day. Then I would be physically with it but not mentally . . .

P   Indeed the first promise of springtime flowers
    Of life in its littleness in its extremity
    For flowers that laugh and sing and cow or coo
    With life do not exist anymore
    If ever before in prehistoric times.

Another small group of children were those with brain-damage of some sort. In most of these there was a history of injury either at birth or later in some accident, but there were also those with no such history whom the psychologist assessed as probably brain-damaged. All these children presented a similar pattern of behaviour: overexuberance, clumsiness, sudden rages, whimpering petulance and aggressiveness. They made normal development in some areas and it was particularly sad that they often knew that they were disabled and tried to cover up by boastfulness or a 'don't care' attitude. One difficulty was that, in their desire to be accepted and to appear to be as good as the others, they fell prey at times to unscrupulous characters who, under the guise of protecting them, manipulated them into performing anti-social acts. Others would maliciously work them up into frenzies whose consequences might be horrifying.

A number of children were epileptic or had epileptic-like attacks. They often showed a low tolerance of frustration and were inclined to be over-active; they seemed almost compelled to climb, even up into the roof girders. The higher they climbed, the greater our anxiety. Often they were highly intelligent children who were very guilty about their behaviour. In time, their fits were controlled by drugs, but this often made life harder for them in other ways, for the fits were often replaced by outbursts of aggression. So, instead of sympathy for the child who had fallen into a fit, the others felt anger and aggression against an attacker, with little concern about his inner feelings. In these cases, alongside continued medication for the epileptic, a long rehabilitation programme was called for; as much for the attacker as for the attacked.

These badly handicapped children often needed a period when each could be the sole concern of one member of the staff. Although this could not be arranged as often as we would have liked, we provided as many of these periods as we could. Any aptitude that these children might have for academic work, even though it were only number and word recognition, gave them status in the eyes of their more advanced fellows who would constitute themselves teachers. It also helped them communicate in some way with one another.

The biggest group was of children who were not grossly abnormal but who were out of sorts with themselves, with their families, or with society at large. Somewhere along the line of their psychosocial development something essential had been missed out. Instead of trust and initiative, there was mistrust. Shame, doubt, and guilt had led to a sense of inferiority in the latency period, just when they were meeting new problems and should have been finding out how to cope with them. Adolescence, reviving all the unresolved difficulties of infancy, found them helpless and going back rather than forward. They seemed incapable of establishing themselves as adults and we could recognize in them what Erikson calls 'identity diffusion' and 'work paralysis'. How were they going to become independent, self-directing adults? In some of them the death of a parent or relative revived their memories of infantile deprivation. At the late age of seventy-five Colette could write: 'In my heart of hearts I blame them for dying, calling them careless, imprudent. How could they deprive me of their company, and so abruptly, how could they think of doing such a thing to me!'

For some of our children it was when they had to leave the safe world of childhood and the primary school; for others, when they had to change from the secondary school to the adult world of competition, that they knew themselves to be inadequate and lost. The difficulty they had in trusting others led them to suspect that they themselves were worthless and empty. They would say to us: 'There is nothing to do, nothing is any good, there is nothing to live for, nothing. . . .' And, while some children might react to these feelings by producing a compliant false personality, or by turning back into masochistic or suicidal behaviour, more out-going young people would show anger and hatred, fighting for recognition by inflicting punishment, and assuaging their guilt by receiving punishment. Many of these children were as capable of loving as of hating, and often experienced the most violent conflict between what they desired to do and what they did.

Unconscious memories of deprivation and rejection often revealed themselves. Stephen would ask for a pencil, and even as one turned to get it for him, he would say: 'I bet it's broken and won't write.' Arthur would begin to ask for materials, then interrupt himself to say: 'No, don't bother, it won't be any good.' In the face of these reactions, the re-establishment of trust became a vital part of our programme to which all else had to be subordinated.

These boys and girls were but young in the actual number of years they had lived, and on occasion had to be treated as really little ones in human relationships. In one of his training papers for clergy, Dr Frank Lake has written: 'The child at three has acquired many permanently imprinted attitudes of expectancy or non-expectancy towards vital relationships – to expect a welcoming face, a rejecting, scornful or angry face, with correspondingly powerful defensive manœuvres to mitigate encounters which promise to be too terrible.' We were not working with the pre-school child, yet had to resort to pre-language communication, and struggle to make the memory of the rejecting scornful face recede before the welcoming face, and back up the message of the good face by consistently sincere behaviour. Confidence and self-confidence grew together, and a smile might also indicate self-acceptance, as at the end of the following conversation when Fred had taken and smoked another boy's cigarettes:

'Well, you know it was me, why don't you punish me?'
'*You think you should be punished?*'
'Of course I do. I took them.'
'*You would feel good if you were punished?*'
'Yes.'
'*At present you feel horrible?*'
'Yes.'
'*Is there anything else that could take away this horrible feeling if you were not punished?*'
'I am not going to say I am sorry!'
'*No.*'
'I could give him my cigarettes when I get some.'

And later . . .

'I gave him my cigarettes. That all right?'
'*Is it all right?*'
(With a smile) 'Yeah.'

A puzzling situation was created by those children who always seemed to be on the receiving end of hostilities and bullying. At first sight they might seem to be quiet and inoffensive, but gradually the very quietness was seen to be hostile, a kind of deep scorn which would not even concern itself with acknowledging the enemy. They could even be reduced to tears, but never formed any relationship through these contacts. In a way, insignificant and faceless as they often seemed, they made their attackers the faceless ones in a way that could not be tolerated. The only way to help these quiet, inoffensive ones (the answers to a teacher's prayer), was to induce them to play out their hostility in open aggression.

We often wondered whether children with psychotic symptoms should live in the same Unit as those who showed psychotic symptoms fleetingly or not at all. It might have been more comfortable for all of us to live without remembering the disintegrating forces in the personality and we were sure that most of us needed rests from the psychotics. But sometimes the psychotic children helped the others. For instance, Brian, a clever eleven-year-old with apparently no inhibitions at all, even of making attacks on the women teachers, showed the greatest tenderness and concern towards Charles, a schizophrenic sixteen-year-old. With everyone else Brian felt himself to be scorned and worthless, but Charles reassured him that he (Brian) was not at the bottom of the barrel. To please and protect Charles he could control his aggression and subordinate his rebelliousness.

We also wondered about the so-called defective children admitted for diagnosis and felt sad about the way they were treated. Usually, they left us just when they had stayed in the Unit long enough to build up relationships with the staff and to show their potential in the school. It seemed to us that, either they should go before strong relationships were formed, or they should be allowed to stay as long as was necessary to consolidate their gains.

When one of these had a long stay, he gained by making educational and social progress, but he gained even more from the fact that the others lost their fear of him and, with it, their wish to mock or bully. Often, as their attitude changed, they, too, benefited by being able to learn something about their own mental processes and understand the reason for their contempt.

Although only some very grave condition, acute or chronic, brought children into our Unit, some of them always seemed remarkably normal. Once they had settled in they showed no sign of psychosis, of disturbance of behaviour, epilepsy, brain-damage, or of other identifiable disorder. They joined neither the bullying nor the bullied, going their own way competently and quietly, though usually not for long, for their stay with us was all too short.

It was seldom that the children, as individuals, were anything but charming. Many of them, including a number of coloured children, had pronounced physical beauty. Many were intelligent, amusing, lively companions, with flashes of creativity and wit. Always, one felt, there was the promise of better things to come. They differed from one another in their behaviour, in their moods, in their capabilities, their loves, their hates. Yet they were alike in their needs and their hopes and, still more important, in their confidence that we would help them overcome the obstacles to fulfilment.

I felt that I could use Colette's words as she looked from her window upon the boys and girls of Paris:

'But I haven't the heart to curse them, my lively sparrows intoxicated by their own chirrupings, my whistling little cobras, my embryo artillerymen, corn-crake-voiced chatterboxes, and maniac trumpeters . . . I cannot spend my time abusing them, because I observe them and by observation make them my own. I do not lay claim to them in a pseudo-maternity which has never come easily to me, but from my window above I recognize in them my own blood, my own race, my own past, my own faults, whether reclaimed by time or aggravated by age . . .'

She might just have been looking down on Sebastian's!